THE MEDITERRANEAN DIET COOKBOOK IN 30 MINUTES

2000 Days | Fast, Nutritious, and Flavorful Recipes for Busy Health-Conscious Individuals | 30-Day Meal Plan Included!

**Theresa R. Campanella**

TABLE OF CONTENTS

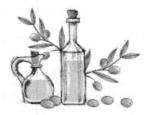

MEDITERRANEAN DIET SHOPPING LIST

STAPLES

Oils
- [ ] Olive Oil
- [ ] Extra-virgin olive oil

Vinegar
- [ ] Balsamic
- [ ] Red wine
- [ ] White wine

A variety of dried herbs & spices
- [ ] Basil
- [ ] Parsley
- [ ] Oregano
- [ ] Cayenne pepper
- [ ] Cinnamon
- [ ] Cloves
- [ ] Cumin
- [ ] Coriander
- [ ] Dill
- [ ] Fennel seed
- [ ] Ginger
- [ ] Rosemary
- [ ] Red and white wine
- [ ] Garlic

MEAT & SEAFOOD

- [ ] Clams
- [ ] Cod
- [ ] Crab meat
- [ ] Halibut
- [ ] Mussels
- [ ] Salmon
- [ ] Scallops
- [ ] Shrimp
- [ ] Tilapia
- [ ] Tuna
- [ ] Chicken breast*
- [ ] Chicken thighs*
- [ ] Lean red meat**

CANNED & PACKAGED

- [ ] Olives
- [ ] Canned Tomatoes

Dried & canned beans
- [ ] Cannellini beans
- [ ] Navy beans
- [ ] Chickpeas
- [ ] Black beans
- [ ] Kidney beans
- [ ] Lentils
- [ ] Canned tuna

Whole Grains
- [ ] Whole grain pasta
- [ ] Bulgur
- [ ] Whole wheat couscous
- [ ] Quinoa
- [ ] Brown rice
- [ ] Barley
- [ ] Faro
- [ ] Polenta
- [ ] Oats
- [ ] Whole wheat bread or pita
- [ ] Whole grain crackers

Nuts & seeds
- [ ] Almonds
- [ ] Hazelnuts
- [ ] Pine nuts
- [ ] Walnuts
- [ ] Cashews
- [ ] Sunflower seeds
- [ ] Sesame seeds

REFRIGERATED

Cheese
- [ ] Cream cheese
- [ ] Feta
- [ ] Goat cheese
- [ ] Mozzarella
- [ ] Parmesan
- [ ] Ricotta
- [ ] Low-fat milk
- [ ] Plain or Greek yogurt
- [ ] Eggs

PRODUCE

- [ ] Apples
- [ ] Artichokes
- [ ] Asparagus
- [ ] Avocado
- [ ] Bananas
- [ ] Beets
- [ ] Bell peppers
- [ ] Berries (all types)
- [ ] Broccoli
- [ ] Brussels sprouts
- [ ] Cabbage
- [ ] Carrots
- [ ] Celery
- [ ] Cherries
- [ ] Cucumbers
- [ ] Dates
- [ ] Eggplant
- [ ] Fennel
- [ ] Figs
- [ ] Grapes
- [ ] Green beans
- [ ] Kiwi
- [ ] Leafy greens
- [ ] Lemons
- [ ] Lettuce
- [ ] Limes
- [ ] Melons
- [ ] Mushrooms
- [ ] Nectarines
- [ ] Onions
- [ ] Oranges
- [ ] Peas
- [ ] Peaches
- [ ] Pears
- [ ] Plums
- [ ] Pomegranate
- [ ] Potatoes
- [ ] Shallots
- [ ] Spinach
- [ ] Squash
- [ ] Tomatoes
- [ ] Zucchini

* In moderation, once to twice per week
** On rare occasions, once to twice monthly

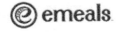 emeals

Credit By Emeals

INTRODUCTION

Welcome to "The Mediterranean Diet in 30 Minutes"! Are you a busy individual looking to adopt a Mediterranean diet but finding it challenging to come up with quick and easy recipes? This book aims to provide you with a wealth of delicious and nutritious meals that can be prepared in 30 minutes or less. Our goal is to make it easier than ever for you to embrace the Mediterranean lifestyle, even with a packed schedule.

In this book, we have curated a diverse range of recipes suitable for beginners. We understand the importance of time and have carefully selected recipes that are bursting with flavor while also being healthy and requiring minimal effort. Even on the busiest days, you don't have to sacrifice flavor or nutrients.

Numerous health advantages of the Mediterranean diet have been widely documented, including better heart health, better control of weight, and general wellbeing. You may enjoy these advantages while eating a broad range of delectable foods by implementing the tenets of the Mediterranean diet into your everyday life.

This book is here to accompany you on your road to a Mediterranean diet, whether you're a committed professional, a parent juggling several commitments, or just someone who values their time. Our aim is to empower you with practical and easy-to-follow recipes that will nourish both your body and your taste buds.

Together, we will explore the world of quick and simple Mediterranean cuisine, guiding you through the process of creating delightful meals in just 30 minutes or less. With our informative, supportive, and passionate approach, you'll be well-prepared to embark on this flavorful and health-conscious adventure.

The Best Diet in The World Is the Mediterranean

According to a U.S. study based on the Best Diet Ranking 2021, this was released.

In the year of COVID, the Mediterranean diet is rated as the greatest diet in the world, surpassing the dash and flexitarian. This was shown by a study based on the best diet rating for 2021 created by the renowned American media outlet "**U.S. News & World Report,**" which is known around the world for producing rankings and consumer advise.

The first-place finishes in five distinct categories—diabetes prevention and treatment, heart protection, healthy eating, plant-based components, and ease of implementation—helped the Mediterranean diet establish its overall dominance.

What if we told you that an American scientist truly researched and organized the Mediterranean diet? Yes, Ancel Keys, an American scientist and physiologist, thoroughly examined and contrasted the diets of the residents of the Mediterranean basin with those of other nations at the start of the 1950s.

The famous Seven Countries Study, managed by Keys, was based on the observation of the eating habits and lifestyles of seven countries (United States, Finland, Netherlands, Italy, Greece, Japan and former

Yugoslavia), with the objective of understanding the effects on the wellbeing of the population, with particular attention paid to the incidence of cardiovascular diseases.

In Northern European countries, milk, potatoes, animal fats, and sweets were the most commonly consumed foods. In the United States, meat, fruit, and sweets were the most commonly consumed foods. In Italy, it was clear that cereals (especially bread and pasta) and wine were widely consumed. In the former Yugoslavia, bread, vegetables, and wine were the most commonly consumed foods.

Keys study showed that a diet focused on cereals, vegetables, fruit, fish, and olive oil was by far superior to the conventional American and northern European diets, which are too high in fats, animal proteins, and sweets.

A Food Pyramid that depicts the amount and frequency of food to be taken throughout the day summarizes the principles of the Mediterranean diet, which is now recognized by **UNESCO** as a universally beneficial intangible.

CHAPTER 1: *Getting Started with the Mediterranean Diet*

Welcome to Chapter 1 of "The Mediterranean Diet in 30 Minutes." This chapter will establish the groundwork for your adventure into the Mediterranean diet by giving you the necessary knowledge and helpful advice to get started on this wholesome and delectable eating style.

Understanding the Mediterranean Diet

We will go into the fundamental ideas and philosophy of the Mediterranean diet in this part. You will learn about the long history, cultural importance, and overall health and wellbeing benefits of this food pattern. We will look into the Mediterranean way of life, emphasizing its focus on seasonal eating, whole, unprocessed foods, and mindful mealtime enjoyment. We'll provide you with useful advice and tactics so you can stick to the Mediterranean diet successfully despite your busy schedule. The Mediterranean diet can be easily incorporated into your everyday routine by learning how to plan meals, buy groceries, organize your kitchen, and save time.

Benefits of the Mediterranean Diet

Here, we'll examine the many advantages the Mediterranean diet has for your health. You'll learn the compelling arguments for why the Mediterranean diet has attracted attention from around the world, including lowering the risk of chronic diseases like heart disease and diabetes, facilitating weight management, and improving cognitive performance.

The Mediterranean Lifestyle

Embracing simplicity and balance: Discover how the Mediterranean lifestyle encourages a balanced approach to food, exercise, and relaxation. We'll discuss the importance of enjoying meals with loved ones, savoring each bite, and practicing mindful eating.

Seasonal and local eating: Learn about the Mediterranean emphasis on fresh, seasonal, and locally sourced ingredients. We'll talk about the advantages of using locally grown fruits and vegetables as well as how to change your menus to take advantage of seasonal products.

Active Living: Learn about the importance of physical activity to general health and wellbeing and the Mediterranean approach to it. From daily walks to engaging in recreational activities, we'll uncover the joy of staying active and its positive impact on your Mediterranean lifestyle.

Characteristics of Mediterranean Diet

The Mediterranean diet is characterized by a number of components that must be consumed each day in precisely calculated amounts in order to achieve a balanced diet that contains all the macronutrients and is distributed as follows: **60% carbs, 25%–30% fats, and 10%–15% proteins.**

3 portions of unrefined grains, such as pasta, rice, and bread, but also spelt or oats, 3 portions of fruit, and 6 portions of vegetables should be consumed each day.

Yogurt and milk can be had daily, while cheese should only be consumed twice per week.

Animal proteins are by far inferior to those found in plants, such as those found in legumes. It is advised to eat fish three to four times per week rather than white meat, which should only be consumed once or twice a week.

The Mediterranean diet allows for a maximum of three servings of fat per day, with a preference for monounsaturated fats, particularly olive oil.

A reduction in sausages, alcohol, white sugar, butter, fatty cheese, white salt, beef and pork, lard, and coffee is part of the Mediterranean diet. Sweets, instead, are allowed on certain occasions.

Traditional Mediterranean Ingredients

- **Vibrant fruits and vegetables**: Discover the colorful array of fruits and vegetables commonly found in Mediterranean cuisine. We'll spotlight particular types, their distinctive flavor qualities, and the health advantages they offer.
- **Whole grains and legumes:** Learn about the wide variety of whole grains and legumes used in Mediterranean cooking. We'll examine the adaptability and health advantages of these mainstays, from hearty whole wheat bread to protein-rich chickpeas.
- **Flavorful herbs and spices:** Delve into the aromatic world of Mediterranean herbs and spices. We'll introduce you to common flavors like oregano, basil, and thyme, as well as special spice combinations that give Mediterranean meals depth and complexity.
- **Olive oil and other healthy fats**: Gain a deeper understanding of olive oil—the liquid gold of the Mediterranean—and how it contributes to both the flavor and health benefits of the diet. We'll also look at additional good sources of fat, like seeds, almonds, and avocados.
- **Mediterranean pantry essentials**: Discover the must-have ingredients that form the backbone of a well-stocked Mediterranean pantry. From canned tomatoes to olives and capers, we'll guide you through building a pantry that supports your Mediterranean cooking endeavors.

The Mediterranean Food Pyramid

- ✓ **Foundation of plant-based foods:** Find out what constitutes the foundation of the Mediterranean diet: an abundance of fruits, vegetables, whole grains, legumes, nuts, and seeds. We'll go through the health advantages of each food type and offer helpful advice on cooking with them.
- ✓ **Healthy fats and oils**: Learn why olive oil, which is high in monounsaturated fatty acids and antioxidants, is preferred in the Mediterranean region. We'll also look at additional good sources of fat and how they support heart health and general wellbeing.
- ✓ **Moderate consumption of fish, poultry, and dairy:** Understand the role of lean proteins such as fish and poultry, as well as the moderate consumption of dairy products, in the Mediterranean diet. We'll provide guidance on selecting high-quality sources and incorporating them into your meals.
- ✓ **Occasional consumption of red meat and sweets:** Explore the balanced approach to red meat and sweets in the Mediterranean diet. We'll discuss portion control, mindful indulgence, and healthier alternatives to enjoy these foods in moderation.

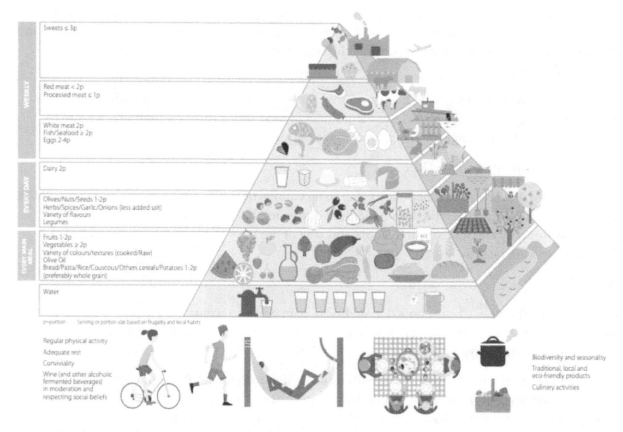

The following text labels appear within the pyramid image:

Sweets ≤ 3p

Red meat < 2p
Processed meat ≤ 1p

White meat 2p
Fish/Seafood ≥ 2p
Eggs 2-4p

Dairy 2p

Olives/Nuts/Seeds 1-2p
Herbs/Spices/Garlic/Onions (less added salt)
Variety of flavours
Legumes

Fruits 1-2p
Vegetables ≥ 2p
Variety of colours/textures (cooked/Raw)
Olive Oil
Bread/Pasta/Rice/Couscous/Others cereals/Potatoes 1-2p
(preferably whole grain)

Water

p=portion   Serving or portion size based on frugality and local habits

Regular physical activity
Adequate rest
Conviviality
Wine (and other alcoholic
fermented beverages)
in moderation and
respecting social beliefs

Biodiversity and seasonality
Traditional, local and
eco-friendly products
Culinary activities

Food pyramid – Credit: International Journal of Enviromental Research and Public Health

What is the food pyramid? It is a visual tool used to convey, in an easy, efficient, and quick manner, which meals should be ingested more frequently during a week and in what amounts. The items listed at the bottom of the pyramid should be taken more frequently and in larger quantities; as one moves up the pyramid toward the top, the relative frequency of intake should decline but not completely disappear.

This pyramid has a major innovation that is evident in the visual representation: there is a third dimension at each level that depicts the environmental component and the particular influence that each food group has on the environment.

A healthy and sustainable diet has been suggested in the new pyramid for both our welfare and the wellbeing of the planet. Maintaining the original Mediterranean model, which, let's not forget, was made up of numerous meals of vegetable origin, it is mostly based on foods of vegetable origin but not exclusively.

Additionally, the Mediterranean diet has advantages for the environment because it promotes a high intake of cereals, fruits, vegetables, and legumes, which require less intensive use of natural resources and produce fewer greenhouse gas emissions than a diet that emphasizes the consumption of meat and animal fats.

The pyramid suggests ingesting legumes once a day in order to increase sustainability, further reducing consumption of processed red meat, cheese, and packaged meals.

This model emphasizes the value of selecting and consuming vegetables and vegetal foods in accordance with their seasonality and, if possible, local availability. Doing so will reduce greenhouse cultivation and the associated environmental impacts, as well as the costs and pollution associated with shipping produce from distant lands.

The biodiversity of the region has long been a priority for the Mediterranean diet, which also emphasizes the value of conviviality and the naturalness of food. With this new upgrade, we aim to increase people's food knowledge and help them make better dinnertime decisions.

Benefits of the Mediterranean Diet

The Mediterranean diet has gained popularity due to its various health benefits. In this part, we will look at the benefits of following a Mediterranean diet for your general health. Understanding these advantages will not only encourage you to adopt this way of life but will also push you to make long-term adjustments for a healthy future.

Heart Health

Reduced risk of heart disease: Learn how the Mediterranean diet's concentration on plant-based foods, healthy fats, and moderate consumption of lean meats helps to maintain cardiovascular health. We'll look at the research that backs up the diet's potential to lower the risk of heart disease.

Lower blood pressure: Discover how the Mediterranean diet, with its emphasis on whole grains, fruits, and vegetables and low salt intake, may aid in the maintenance of healthy blood pressure levels. We'll talk about how particular nutrients and meals affect blood pressure management.

- Lower cholesterol levels: Investigate the Mediterranean diet's effect in establishing healthy cholesterol profiles. We'll go through how include monounsaturated fats, fiber-rich foods, and omega-3 fatty acids in your diet might improve your lipid profile.

Weight Management

Sustainable weight loss: Understand how the Mediterranean diet's nutrient-dense, whole-food approach can support weight loss and weight management. We'll talk about portion management, mindful eating, and the delight that comes from experimenting with different flavors and textures.

Long-term weight maintenance: Learn about the Mediterranean diet's sustainable character, which increases the likelihood of individuals maintaining their weight reduction in the long run. We'll look at the diet's satiating capabilities as well as its capacity to produce a healthy body composition.

Visceral fat reduction: Learn how the Mediterranean diet can help decrease unhealthy visceral fat, which is linked to an elevated risk of chronic illnesses. We'll go through the precise dietary elements that lead to this beneficial impact.

Brain Health

Investigate the evidence associating the Mediterranean diet with increased cognitive performance and memory preservation. We'll talk about how antioxidants, omega-3 fatty acids, and other nutrients can help with brain health.

- **the risk of neurodegenerative disorders:** Learn how the anti-inflammatory qualities and protective elements in the Mediterranean diet might help lower the risk of neurodegenerative diseases like Alzheimer's and Parkinson's. We'll focus on certain meals and nutrients that are important for brain health.

Mental well-being: Learn about the Mediterranean diet's influence on mental well-being and its potential to lower the risk of depression and anxiety. We'll look at the relationship between gut health and mental health, as well as how food may help maintain a healthy gut flora.

Overall Health and Longevity

Reduced risk of chronic diseases: Reduced risk of chronic illnesses: Discover how the Mediterranean diet's anti-inflammatory, nutrient-rich foods can help lower the risk of chronic diseases such as type 2 diabetes, some malignancies, and metabolic syndrome. We'll go over the scientific data that backs up these relationships.

Anti-aging properties: Explore the potential anti-aging effects of the Mediterranean diet. We'll discuss the role of antioxidants, polyphenols, and other bioactive compounds in protecting against oxidative stress and promoting cellular health.

Enhanced longevity: Discover the link between the Mediterranean diet and increased life expectancy. We'll explore the lifestyle factors, nutritional components, and disease prevention mechanisms that contribute to a longer, healthier life.

Quick Tips for Success

The Mediterranean diet is a way of life steeped in centuries-old traditions and a strong connection to nature and community. Adopting a new dietary habit might be daunting at times, but with the appropriate tactics and mentality, you can fit the Mediterranean diet into your daily routine with ease.

Start Slow and Gradual

Gradual transition: Ease into the Mediterranean diet by gradually incorporating its principles into your meals. Start by adding more fruits, vegetables, and whole grains to your plate and gradually reducing processed foods.

Tiny adjustments, huge impact: Don't try to make an overnight transformational shift; instead, concentrate on creating tiny, lasting changes. You may create enduring habits and boost your chances of long-term success by using this strategy.

Accept Plant-Based Meals

Make veggies the star of the show: Include a range of vibrant vegetables in all of your meals. Try out various cooking techniques and tastes to make them appetizing and fun.

Legumes and whole grains: Include legumes like lentils, chickpeas, and beans in your diet together with nutritious grains like quinoa, brown rice, and whole wheat bread. They keep you full while supplying vital nutrients and fiber.

Choose healthy fats: Increase your intake of olive oil, avocados, almonds, and seeds, which are high in monounsaturated fats and good for your heart. Limit your intake of saturated and trans fats contained in processed meals.

Choose Lean Proteins

Select lean sources: Prioritize lean proteins such as fish, poultry, and plant-based options like tofu and tempeh. These provide essential amino acids without excessive saturated fat.

Moderate red meat consumption: Enjoy red meat occasionally and opt for lean cuts. Limit processed meats due to their association with health risks.

Include dairy and dairy alternatives: Incorporate low-fat dairy products or their plant-based alternatives, like unsweetened almond or soy milk, into your diet for calcium and protein.

Flavor with Herbs and Spices

Explore Mediterranean herbs by experimenting with basil, oregano, rosemary, and thyme. Add flavor to your food using herbs and spices. These herbs not only enhance flavor but may also have health advantages.

Spice it up: Add depth and complexity to your foods by using spices such as turmeric, cumin, paprika, and cinnamon. Discover their distinct tastes as well as their possible health-promoting benefits.

Reduce sodium intake: Rely on herbs, spices, and other flavor enhancers to reduce your reliance on added salt, promoting better heart health.

Practice Mindful Eating

Slow down and savor: Take the time to enjoy your meals and savor each bite. Eating mindfully helps you recognize when you are full and prevents overeating.

Portion control: Be aware of portion sizes and listen to your body's hunger and fullness cues. This mindful approach to eating promotes a healthy relationship with food.

Engage all senses: Appreciate the aroma, appearance, and texture of your meals. Engaging all your senses enhances your eating experience and satisfaction.

CHAPTER 2: *Essential Ingredients and Pantry Staples*

Before we get into the recipes, it's important to understand the fundamental elements that make up the Mediterranean diet. In this chapter, we'll look at the essential components of a well-stocked Mediterranean pantry to ensure you have everything you need to make delectable cuisine.

Seasonal fruits and vegetables

Fresh produce and seasonal fruits are important components of the Mediterranean diet since they are high in vitamins, minerals, and antioxidants. We'll talk about how important it is to include a range of fresh fruits and vegetables in your Mediterranean-inspired meals. We'll also go through how to choose, store, and use these healthy items.

Fresh produce plays an important role in the Mediterranean diet, delivering a wealth of health advantages.

The Mediterranean diet emphasizes the consumption of fresh, whole foods, particularly fruits and vegetables. Let's investigate the benefits of including fresh vegetables in your diet:

- ✓ **Nutrient density**: Fresh fruits and vegetables are full of vital elements such as vitamins, minerals, and dietary fiber. This is known as their "nutrient density." They include a wide variety of micronutrients that support overall health and wellbeing.
- ✓ **Chronic diseases**: Fruits and vegetables are abundant in antioxidants, which aid in the body's fight against oxidative stress and inflammation. These ingredients support a strong immune system and aid in preventing chronic diseases.
- ✓ **Hydration and fiber**: Fruits and vegetables with high water content will help you stay hydrated. They also include a lot of dietary fiber, which aids in digestion and increases feelings of fullness.
- ✓ **Low Calorie, High Volume**: The majority of fruits and vegetables have a high volume while containing little calories. This implies that you may eat large servings without sacrificing your calorie intake.

Seasonal Fruits and Their Health Benefits

Eating fruits in season not only adds taste to your meals, but it also assures that you're getting the freshest and most nutrient-dense food available. The availability of seasonal vegetables has a great impact on the diet in the Mediterranean area. Here are several seasonal fruits and their associated health benefits:

1. Citrus Fruits: Citrus fruits, including oranges, lemons, and grapefruits, are high in vitamin C, which helps with immunological function and collagen formation. They also contain flavonoids, which are potent antioxidants with anti-inflammatory effects.

2. Berries: Antioxidants and phytochemicals abound in strawberries, blueberries, and raspberries. These colorful fruits improve brain function, defend against oxidative damage, and help the heart.

3. Stone Fruits: Peaches, plums, and apricots are not only tasty but also high in dietary fiber and vitamins A and C. They promote healthy skin, eyesight, and immunological function.

4. Melons: Watermelons, cantaloupes, and honeydews are hydrating fruits with a high-water content. They are also high in vitamins A and C, as well as electrolytes like potassium.

Recommended Fruits and Vegetables for Mediterranean-Inspired Meals

While the Mediterranean area has a broad variety of fruits and vegetables, we'll focus on some of the more popular and flexible selections. You'll learn how to use these delectable items to add a burst of freshness and nutritional value to your meals.

Here are some examples of versatile fruits and vegetables used in Mediterranean cooking:

1. **Tomato**: Tomatoes are a common ingredient in Mediterranean cuisine and may be found in salads, sauces, and roasted meals.

2. **Leafy Greens** like spinach, kale, and arugula are high in vitamins, minerals, and antioxidants. They're great in salads, sautés, and as the basis for a variety of Mediterranean-inspired meals.

3. **Eggplant**: This versatile vegetable may be grilled, roasted, or included in stews and dips such as baba ganoush.

4. **Zucchini and Squash**: Grilling, sautéing, or spiralizing zucchini and summer squash into "zoodles" as a lighter alternative to pasta.

5. **Bell Peppers:** Bell peppers add vibrant color and flavor to Mediterranean recipes. They can be used in salads, stir-fries, or stuffed with a variety of fillings.

Whole Grains and Legumes

Whole grains and legumes are important components of the Mediterranean diet because they are high in complex carbs, fiber, protein, and critical minerals. We'll talk about how to include healthy grains and legumes in your Mediterranean-inspired dishes.

Health Benefits of Whole Grains and Legumes

Including whole grains and legumes in your diet offers a myriad of health benefits. Let's take a look at some of them:

- ✓ **Dietary Fiber:** Whole grains and legumes are excellent sources of dietary fiber, which promotes healthy digestion, regulates blood sugar levels, and helps maintain a feeling of fullness.
- ✓ **Nutrient Richness:** Whole grains and legumes provide an array of essential nutrients, including B vitamins, iron, magnesium, and potassium. These nutrients support energy production, nerve function, and overall well-being.
- ✓ **Heart Health:** The soluble fiber found in whole grains and legumes helps reduce cholesterol levels, lowers the risk of heart disease, and supports cardiovascular health.
- ✓ **Weight Management**: Due to their high fiber content and satisfying nature, whole grains and legumes can contribute to weight management by promoting feelings of fullness and reducing overeating.

Varieties of Whole Grains and Legumes

There are numerous varieties of whole grains and legumes to explore and enjoy. Here are some popular options:

1. **Whole Grains:**

Brown rice: is a versatile grain that can be used in pilafs, stir-fries, and side dishes.

- **Quinoa:** A complete protein source that can be used as a base for salads, grain bowls, or as a substitute for rice.

- **Bulgur:** A quick-cooking grain used in dishes like tabbouleh and pilafs.

Whole wheat pasta: is a nutritious alternative to traditional pasta, providing more fiber and nutrients.

2. **Legumes:**

- **Chickpeas:** Versatile legumes used in hummus, stews, salads, and roasted as a crunchy snack.

- are Quick-cooking legumes available in various colors and commonly used in soups, stews, and salads.

- **Black beans**: A protein-rich legume that can be used in wraps, tacos, soups, or as a base for veggie burgers.

- **Cannellini beans:** Creamy beans used in Mediterranean dishes like minestrone soup and bean salads.

Incorporating Whole Grains and Legumes into Your Diet

Here are some practical tips for incorporating whole grains and legumes into your Mediterranean-inspired meals:

1. Experiment with different whole grains and legumes to discover new flavors and textures.

2. Replace refined grains with whole grain options like whole wheat bread, whole grain cereals, and brown rice.

3. Add cooked legumes to salads, soups, and stews, or use them as a protein-rich base for vegetarian meals.

4. Use whole grain flours in baking recipes to increase the nutritional value of bread, muffins, and pancakes

Healthy Fats and Oils

Healthy fats and oils are important components of the Mediterranean diet because they provide needed nutrients, taste, and culinary diversity. In this section, we'll look at how to include healthy fats and oils in your Mediterranean-inspired recipes. We'll talk about their health advantages, different varieties, and how to include them in your meals.

Health Benefits of Healthy Fats and Oils

Contrary to popular belief, not all fats are detrimental to your health. Healthy fats and oils offer numerous benefits and are an essential component of the Mediterranean diet. Let's explore their health benefits:

✓ **Heart Health**: Healthy fats, such as monounsaturated fats and omega-3 fatty acids, can help lower bad cholesterol levels, reduce inflammation, and promote heart health.

- ✓ **Nutrient Absorption**: Certain vitamins, such as vitamins A, D, E, and K, are fat-soluble, meaning they require the presence of dietary fats for optimal absorption in the body.
- ✓ **Brain Function**: Omega-3 fatty acids found in fatty fish and plant-based sources like flaxseeds and walnuts are beneficial for brain health, cognition, and mood regulation.
- ✓ **Satiety and Flavor:** Including healthy fats in your meals enhances satiety, helping you feel fuller for longer. Fats also contribute to the flavor, texture, and overall enjoyment of your dishes.

Types of Healthy Fats and Oils

Here are some healthy fats and oils commonly used in the Mediterranean diet:

1. Extra virgin olive oil: An essential component of the Mediterranean diet, extra virgin olive oil has anti-inflammatory, antioxidant, and high levels of monounsaturated fatty acids. It is perfect for low-heat cooking, sautéing, and dressings.

2. Avocado: An excellent source of beneficial monounsaturated fats is found in the fruit of the avocado. On toast, in salads, or as a creamy addition to smoothies, it is delicious when sliced.

3. Nuts and Seeds: Nutrient-dense sources of healthy fats include almonds, walnuts, flaxseeds, chia seeds, and sesame seeds. They can be eaten as snacks, included in salads or yogurt, or used as garnishes on a variety of foods.

4. Fatty Fish: Fish high in omega-3 fatty acids include salmon, mackerel, sardines, and trout. For best results, incorporate them into your diet on a weekly basis.

Flavorful Herbs and Spices

Herbs and spices are the hidden elements that give Mediterranean recipes depth, scent, and taste. We'll look at the herbs and spices that are widely used in Mediterranean cooking. Learn how these natural spices may improve the flavor of your dishes, provide health benefits, and make your cooking experience more joyful.

Exploring Mediterranean Herbs and Spices

Mediterranean cuisine is renowned for its abundant use of herbs and spices, which contribute to its vibrant and enticing flavors. Here are some popular herbs and spices you'll find in Mediterranean cooking:

1. Basil: Known for its sweet and slightly peppery flavor, basil is a versatile herb used in various Mediterranean dishes, particularly Italian cuisine. It pairs well with tomatoes, cheese, and Mediterranean vegetables.

2. Oregano: With its robust and earthy flavor, oregano is a staple herb in Mediterranean cooking. It adds depth to tomato-based sauces, roasted vegetables, grilled meats, and Greek-inspired dishes.

3. Rosemary: Rosemary has a distinct pine-like aroma and a slightly minty, woody flavor. It pairs well with roasted potatoes, lamb, chicken, and bread. Its flavor intensifies when heated, making it a popular choice for Mediterranean roasted dishes.

4. Thyme: Thyme is a fragrant herb with a slightly floral and earthy flavor. It complements various Mediterranean dishes, including roasted vegetables, grilled fish, soups, and stews.

5. Garlic: Garlic is a fundamental ingredient in Mediterranean cuisine, adding depth and pungency to dishes. It can be used fresh, roasted, or minced, enhancing the flavors of pasta sauces, roasted meats, and vegetable dishes.

6. Paprika: Paprika is a spice made from ground red bell peppers or chili peppers, providing a sweet, smoky, and slightly spicy flavor. It adds a rich, earthy taste to stews, grilled meats, and roasted vegetables.

7. Cumin: Cumin has a warm, earthy, and slightly nutty flavor, commonly used in Mediterranean spice blends and Middle Eastern dishes. It adds depth to roasted vegetables, grains, and legumes.

8. Turmeric: Turmeric has a vibrant golden color and a warm, slightly bitter flavor. It is often used in Mediterranean-inspired curry dishes, rice dishes, roasted vegetables, and marinades.

Essential Kitchen Tools

Equipping your kitchen with the right tools can greatly enhance your experience with the Mediterranean diet. We'll explore the essential kitchen tools that will make meal preparation more efficient and enjoyable. These tools will help you save time, achieve desired cooking techniques, and create delicious Mediterranean dishes with ease.

Must-Have Kitchen Tools for Mediterranean Cooking

1. Chef's Knife: A sharp and versatile chef's knife is an essential tool for every cook. It allows you to slice, dice, and chop ingredients with precision, making meal preparation a breeze.

2. Cutting Board: Choose a sturdy cutting board that provides ample space for chopping fruits, vegetables, and herbs. Opt for a cutting board made of wood or plastic, as they are easier to clean and maintain.

3. Measuring Cups and Spoons: Accurate measurements are crucial for achieving the right balance of flavors in your Mediterranean recipes. Invest in a set of measuring cups and spoons to ensure consistent results.

4. Mixing Bowls: A variety of mixing bowls in different sizes will come in handy for preparing marinades, dressings, and tossing salads. Choose bowls made of stainless steel or glass for durability and easy cleaning.

5. Non-Stick Skillet: A non-stick skillet is ideal for cooking Mediterranean dishes with less oil and easier cleanup. It allows for even heat distribution and prevents ingredients from sticking to the pan.

6. Baking Sheet: A baking sheet or sheet pan is essential for roasting vegetables, preparing homemade bread, or baking Mediterranean-inspired desserts. Look for a sturdy baking sheet with a non-stick surface for best results.

7. Blender or Food Processor: A blender or food processor is useful for preparing smoothies, sauces, dips, and dressings. It helps you achieve a smooth texture and blend ingredients effortlessly.

8. Grater or Zester: A grater or zester allows you to grate or zest ingredients like cheese, citrus fruits, garlic, and ginger, adding flavors and textures to your Mediterranean dishes.

9. Salad Spinner: A salad spinner helps you wash and dry leafy greens and herbs, ensuring they are clean and ready to be used in salads or other dishes.

10. Citrus Juicer: Freshly squeezed citrus juice adds a vibrant and tangy flavor to many Mediterranean recipes. A citrus juicer Serves extracting juice from lemons, limes, and oranges a breeze.

CHAPTER 3: *Quick and Easy Breakfasts*

Starting the day with a nutritious and tasty breakfast establishes the foundation for a balanced Mediterranean diet. In this chapter, we'll look at several quick and simple breakfast alternatives that are full of flavor, nutrition, and Mediterranean-inspired ingredients. These meals will keep you energized and satiated until your next meal, all while fitting into your hectic schedule.

Energizing Smoothies and Bowls

Smoothies and smoothie bowls are an excellent way to start the day with a healthy dose of vitamins, minerals, and antioxidants. This section will walk you through the steps of making revitalizing smoothies and smoothie bowls with Mediterranean ingredients and flavor combinations.

This sub-chapter's recipes are intended to give you a healthy and delightful start to your day. These stimulating smoothies and smoothie bowls can help you embrace the Mediterranean morning lifestyle, whether you choose a refreshing fruit-based smoothie or a creamy and protein-rich choice.

By exploring the dishes in this chapter, you'll be able to start your mornings with tasty and nutritious Mediterranean-inspired breakfasts that are quick to make.

Berry Blast Smoothie	Protein-Packed Almond Butter Smoothie

 10' 2   10' 2

Ingredients:

1 cup mixed berries (strawberries, blueberries, raspberries)
1 cup spinach
1 tablespoon honey
1 cup almond milk
1 cup Greek yogurt

1. In a blender, combine the mixed berries, Greek yogurt, spinach, honey, and almond milk.

2. Blend on high speed until smooth and creamy.

Nutritional Information (per serving):

Kcal	Carbs	Protein	Fat	Sugar	Fiber
124	3g	5g	3g	15g	2g

Ingredients:

2 tablespoons almond butter
1 cup Greek yogurt
1 ripe banana
1 cup almond milk
1/2 teaspoon cinnamon
Ice cubes (optional)

1. In a blender, combine the almond butter, Greek yogurt, banana, almond milk, and cinnamon.

2. Blend until smooth and creamy. If desired, add ice cubes and blend again for a chilled smoothie.

3. Pour into glasses and serve.

Nutritional Information (per serving):

Kcal	Carbs	Protein	Fat	Sugar	Fiber
150	14g	6g	7g	10g	2g

Savory Egg Dishes

Eggs are versatile and nutritious, making them a perfect ingredient for quick and satisfying Mediterranean Breakfasts. We'll explore savory egg dishes that are packed with flavors and nutrients to fuel your day.

Baked Eggs with Cottage Cheese	Mediterranean Egg and Spinach Muffins

 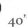 40" 2

  20' 6

Ingredients:

½ medium avocado
3 large eggs
Pinch of sea salt
1 tablespoon. Sliced jalapenos
4 tablespoons Cottage cheese
3 tablespoon Tajin seasoning
1 tablespoon Extra-virgin olive oil
1 tablespoon Smoked paprika

1 tablespoon Onion powder
½ tablespoon garlic powder
¼ cup blended grated cheese
3 ounces chopped broccoli
3 ounces Cauliflower
5 ounces Zucchini diced
1/2 medium green bell pepper diced

1. First, preheat the oven to 400 degrees F.

2. In a large pan, spread diced zucchini, cauliflower, broccoli, and green bell pepper and drizzle with olive oil.

3. Add onion powder, garlic powder, sea salt, and paprika and toss to coat. Layer evenly.

4. Bake for 10 to 15 minutes, or until brown. Take the vegetables out and top with the blended grated cheese.

5. Slice the avocado in half and remove the seed. Place the vegetables inside the hole of the avocado.

6. Add the vegetable mixture and crack the eggs on top of the mixture. Bake for 10 minutes.

7. Top with jalapenos, cottage cheese, tajin

Nutritional Information (per serving):

Kcal	Carbs	Protein	Fat	Sugar	Fiber
170	8g	10g	12g	3g	3g

Ingredients:

6 large eggs
1/2 cup baby spinach, chopped
1/4 cup diced red bell pepper

1/4 cup crumbled feta cheese
1/4 teaspoon dried oregano
Salt and pepper to taste

1. Preheat the oven to 180°C (350°F) and grease a muffin tin.

2. In a bowl, whisk together the eggs, chopped baby spinach, diced red bell pepper, crumbled feta cheese, dried oregano, salt, and pepper.

3. Fill each cup in the muffin tray about 3/4 full with the egg mixture.

4. Bake the egg muffins in the preheated oven for 15-20 minutes, or until the tops are firm and just beginning to turn brown.

5. Take them out of the oven and allow them to cool before removing them from the pan.

6. Serve warmly or store in the fridge for later.

Nutritional Information (per serving):

Kcal	Carbs	Protein	Fat	Sugar	Fiber
135	1g	10g	9g	1g	1g

Mediterranean Egg and Avocado Toast

 10' 2

Ingredients:

2 slices whole-grain bread	1/4 teaspoon red pepper flakes (optional)
2 large eggs	Salt and pepper to taste
1 avocado, mashed	
Fresh cilantro leaves for garnish	

1. Toast the slices of whole-grain bread until crispy.

2. Spread the mashed avocado evenly on each slice of toast. In a skillet, fry the eggs to your preferred doneness. Place one fried egg on top of each slice of avocado toast.

3. Sprinkle with red pepper flakes (if using) and season with salt and pepper. Garnish with fresh cilantro leaves and serve immediately.

Nutritional Information (per serving):

Kcal	Carbs	Protein	Fat	Sugar	Fiber
115	8g	5g	7g	1g	2g

Overnight Oats and Chia Puddings

Overnight oats and chia puddings are convenient make-ahead breakfast options that require minimal effort in the morning

Blueberry Overnight Oats

 15' 2

Ingredients:

1/2 cup rolled oats	1 tablespoon honey or maple syrup
1/2 cup milk (dairy or plant-based)	1/2 teaspoon vanilla extract
Optional toppings: additional fresh blueberries, sliced almonds, or shredded coconut	1/4 cup fresh blueberries
	1/4 cup Greek yogurt
	1 tablespoon chia seeds

1. In a jar or container, combine rolled oats, milk, Greek yogurt, chia seeds, honey or maple syrup, and vanilla extract. Stir well to combine.

2. Add fresh blueberries and gently mix them into the oat mixture.

3. Cover the jar or container and refrigerate overnight or for at least 4 hours.

4. In the morning, give the mixture a stir and add optional toppings such as fresh blueberries, sliced almonds, or shredded coconut.

5. Enjoy the blueberry overnight oats chilled.

Nutritional Information (per serving):

Kcal	Carbs	Protein	Fat	Sugar	Fiber
115	17g	4g	3g	7g	2g

Vanilla Almond Chia Pudding

 15' 2

Ingredients:

1/4 cup chia seeds
1 cup milk (dairy or plant-based)
1 tablespoon honey or maple syrup

1/2 teaspoon vanilla extract
Sliced almonds for topping

1. Chia seeds, milk, honey or maple syrup, and vanilla essence should all be combined in a bowl. To make sure the chia seeds are dispersed equally, stir thoroughly.

2. Stir the mixture once more to avoid clumping after letting it settle for 5 minutes.

3. Wrap the bowl in plastic and chill for at least two hours or overnight.

4. When ready to serve, give the chia pudding a stir to loosen it up.

5. Divide the pudding into serving bowls or jars and sprinkle with sliced almonds.

6. Enjoy the vanilla almond chia pudding chilled.

Nutritional Information (per serving):

Kcal	Carbs	Protein	Fat	Sugar	Fiber
150	13g	5g	9g	7g	5g

Quick Bread and Muffin Recipes

Lemon Bleberry Bread

 15' 50 min

Ingredients:

1 1/2 cups all-purpose flour
1 teaspoon baking powder
1/2 teaspoon baking soda
1/4 teaspoon salt
1/2 cup unsalted butter, softened

2 large eggs
1/2 cup Greek yogurt
Zest of 1 lemon
1 tablespoon lemon juice
1 cup fresh blueberries
3/4 cup granulated sugar

1. Preheat the oven to 350°F (175°C). Grease a loaf pan and set it aside.

2. Combine the flour, baking powder, baking soda, and salt in a medium bowl.

3. Combine the softened butter and sugar in a separate, big bowl and beat until frothy.

4. After adding the Greek yogurt, lemon juice, and lemon zest, beat in each egg one at a time.

5. Stirring until just blended, gradually add the dry ingredients to the wet components.

6. Add the fresh blueberries and gently mix in.

7. Spoon the batter into the loaf pan that has been prepped and level the top with a spatula.

8. Bake for 50 to 60 minutes, or until a toothpick inserted in the center of the cake comes out clean. Remove the bread from the oven and let it cool in the pan for 10 minutes.

Nutritional Information (per serving):

Kcal	Carbs	Protein	Fat	Sugar	Fiber
565	80g	10g	26g	42g	2g

Apple Cinnamon Muffins

 15' 20' 4

Ingredients:

1 1/2 cups all-purpose flour

1/2 cup granulated sugar

2 teaspoons baking powder

1 teaspoon ground cinnamon

1/4 teaspoon salt

1/2 cup unsalted butter, melted

1/2 cup milk (dairy or plant-based)

2 large eggs

1 teaspoon vanilla extract

1 cup grated apple (about 1 medium-sized apple)

1. Set the oven temperature to 375°F (190°C). Paper muffin liners should be used to line a muffin pan.

2. Combine the flour, sugar, baking soda, cinnamon, and salt in a large bowl.

3. Combine the melted butter, milk, eggs, and vanilla extract in another dish.

4. Mix the dry ingredients briefly after adding the liquid components.

5. Stir the grated apple into the mixture until it is thoroughly combined.

6. Distribute the batter equally among the muffin tins, filling each one approximately two-thirds full.

7. Bake for 18 to 20 minutes, or until a toothpick inserted in the middle of the cake comes out clean.

8. Remove the muffins from the oven and allow them to cool in the tin for 5 minutes, then transfer them to a wire rack to cool completely.

Nutritional Information (per serving):

Kcal	Carbs	Protein	Fat	Sugar	Fiber
535	66g	9g	26g	29g	2g

Cheddar Herb Muffins

 15' 20' 4/6

Ingredients:

2 cups all-purpose flour

2 teaspoons baking powder

1/2 teaspoon baking soda

1/2 teaspoon salt

1/2 teaspoon dried thyme

1/2 teaspoon dried rosemary

1/2 teaspoon dried oregano

1/4 teaspoon garlic powder

1/4 teaspoon onion powder

1/4 teaspoon black pepper

2 cups shredded cheddar cheese

1 cup milk (dairy or plant-based)

1/2 cup unsalted butter, melted

1/2 cup plain Greek yogurt

3 large eggs

1. Preheat the oven to 375°F (190°C). Line a muffin tin with paper liners and set aside.

2. In a large bowl, whisk together the flour, baking powder, baking soda, salt, dried thyme, dried rosemary, dried oregano, garlic powder, onion powder, and black pepper.

3. Combine the dry ingredients by thoroughly incorporating the shredded cheddar cheese.

4. Combine the milk, melted butter, Greek yogurt, and eggs in another bowl.

5. Mix the dry ingredients briefly after adding the liquid components. Avoid overmixing. Distribute the batter evenly among the muffin tins, filling each one approximately two-thirds full.

6. Bake for 18 to 20 minutes, or until a toothpick inserted in the middle of the cake comes out clean. After removing the muffins from the oven, let them rest for five minutes in the pan before moving them to a wire rack to finish cooling.

Nutritional Information (per serving):

Kcal	Carbs	Protein	Fat	Sugar	Fiber
758	55g	27g	47g	4g	2g

Mediterranean Bruschetta

 20' 6

Ingredients:

1 French baguette, sliced
2 tablespoons extra-virgin olive oil
2 cloves garlic, halved
1 cup cherry tomatoes, diced
1/2 cup Kalamata olives, pitted and chopped

1/4 cup fresh basil leaves, chopped
2 tablespoons red onion, finely chopped
2 tablespoons balsamic vinegar
Salt and pepper to taste

1. Preheat the oven to 375°F (190°C).

2. Arrange the baguette slices on a baking sheet and brush each slice with olive oil.

3. Toast the baguette slices in the oven for 8-10 minutes, or until golden and crisp.

4. Rub the halved garlic cloves over one side of each toasted baguette slice.

5. In a bowl, combine the cherry tomatoes, Kalamata olives, fresh basil, red onion, and balsamic vinegar.

6. Season with salt and pepper to taste, and mix well.

7. Spoon the tomato mixture onto the garlic-rubbed side of each baguette slice. Serve immediately, and enjoy!

Nutritional Information (per serving):

Kcal	Carbs	Protein	Fat	Sugar	Fiber
260	35g	6g	10g	3g	2g

Fresh Fruit Parfaits and Yogurt Bowls

Fresh fruit parfaits and yogurt bowls are not only visually appealing but also nutritious and refreshing. These recipes are not only quick to prepare but also packed with vitamins, minerals, and antioxidants.

Mixed Berry Parfait

 10' 2

Ingredients:

1 cup Greek yogurt
1 cup mixed berries (such as strawberries, blueberries, and raspberries)

1/4 cup granola
1 tablespoon honey or maple syrup (optional

1. In a glass or bowl, layer half of the Greek yogurt.

2. Add a layer of mixed berries on top of the yogurt.

3. Sprinkle a layer of granola over the berries.

4. Repeat the layers with the remaining yogurt, berries, and granola.

5. Drizzle honey or maple syrup on top for added sweetness if desired.

6. Serve immediately and enjoy!

Nutritional Information (per serving):

Kcal	Carbs	Protein	Fat	Sugar	Fiber
81	8g	4g	3g	8g	1g

Tropical Yogurt Bowl

 10' 1

Ingredients:

1 cup Greek yogurt
1/2 cup chopped pineapple
1/2 cup sliced mango
1/4 cup shredded coconut

2 tablespoons chopped nuts (such as almonds or walnuts)
1 tablespoon chia seeds
1 tablespoon honey or maple syrup (optional)

1. In a bowl, place the Greek yogurt as the base.

2. Arrange the chopped pineapple and sliced mango on top of the yogurt.

3. Sprinkle shredded coconut, chopped nuts, and chia seeds over the fruits.

4. Drizzle honey or maple syrup on top for added sweetness if desired.

5. Mix all the ingredients together before eating, or enjoy each ingredient separately.

Nutritional Information (per serving):

Kcal	Carbs	Protein	Fat	Sugar	Fiber
163	13g	6g	10g	9g	2.6g

Mango Coconut Chia Pudding

 10' 1

Ingredients:

1/4 cup chia seeds
1 cup coconut milk
1 ripe mango, diced
1 tablespoon honey or maple syrup

Toppings: shredded coconut, sliced almonds, fresh mint leaves

1. In a jar or bowl, combine chia seeds and coconut milk.

2. Stir well to mix and let it sit for 5 minutes.

3. Stir the mixture again to prevent clumping of the chia seeds.

4. Cover the jar or bowl and refrigerate for at least 2 hours or overnight until the mixture thickens into a pudding-like consistency.

5. In a serving glass or bowl, layer diced mango and chia pudding.

6. Drizzle honey or maple syrup over the layers.

7. Top with shredded coconut, sliced almonds, and fresh mint leaves.

Nutritional Information (per serving):

Kcal	Carbs	Protein	Fat	Sugar	Fiber
304	23g	5g	23g	14g	7g

CHAPTER 4: *Speedy Salads and Sides*

In Chapter 4 of "The Mediterranean Diet in 30 Minutes," we look at some colorful and nourishing salads and straightforward vegetable side dishes that are quick and simple to make. These dishes are created to go with your main courses and give your meals a burst of flavor and freshness. This chapter includes recipes for both savory side dishes and light, refreshing salads.

These meals highlight the adaptability and health advantages of Mediterranean foods, from bright salad recipes packed with colorful veggies, grains, and legumes to easy and tasty roasted vegetables. Each dish takes only a short amount of time to prepare and is carefully designed to create a harmony of tastes, textures, and nutritional value.

The Mediterranean Diet serves as the basis for these recipes, which place an emphasis on using fresh fruit, healthy fats, whole grains, and flavorful herbs and spices to make delectable dishes that will nourish and satisfy you.

Vibrant Salad Recipes
Salads are a delightful way to incorporate fresh, nutritious ingredients into your Mediterranean diet. This sub-chapter presents a collection of vibrant salad recipes that are bursting with flavors, colors, and textures. These dishes will up your salad game and leave you feeling satiated and fed. They range from robust grain-based salads to refreshing vegetable medleys.

These colorful salad dishes are not only easy to make but also full of vital nutrients, making them the ideal option for a nutritious and well-balanced dinner. You'll discover a number of selections to fit your taste preferences, whether you're searching for a light lunch, a cool side dish, or a colorful appetizer.

These salads, which range from the Mediterranean Quinoa Salad with its delightful combination of grains, vegetables, and feta cheese to the light Greek Salad with its zingy lemon-herb dressing and the traditional Caprese Salad with its decadent mingling of tomatoes, mozzarella, and basil, are sure to tantalize your taste buds and enliven your table.

These dishes are designed to be quick and simple to prepare, so you can enjoy a colorful and filling salad right away

Caprese Salad with Balsamic Glaze

 10' 2

Ingredients:

2 large tomatoes, sliced	2 tablespoons balsamic glaze
8 ounces fresh mozzarella cheese, sliced	2 tablespoons extra-virgin olive oil
Fresh basil leaves	Salt and pepper to taste

1. Alternately arrange the tomato and mozzarella slices on a dish.

2. Sandwich thin slices of tomato and mozzarella with fresh basil.

3. Drizzle the salad with the olive oil and balsamic glaze. To taste, add salt and pepper to the food.

Nutritional Information per Serving:

Kcal	Carbs	Protein	Fat	Sugar	Fiber
235	9g	10g	17g	5g	1g

Mediterranean Quinoa Salad

 10' 2

Ingredients:

1 cup quinoa	1/4 cup Kalamata olives, pitted and halved
2 cups vegetable broth	1/4 cup crumbled feta cheese
1 cucumber, diced	2 tablespoons fresh parsley, chopped
1 bell pepper, diced	
1/2 red onion, thinly sliced	Juice of 1 lemon
1 cup cherry tomatoes, halved	2 tablespoons extra-virgin olive oil
Salt and pepper to taste	

1. Rinse the quinoa under cold water and drain.

2. Bring the vegetable broth to a boil in a saucepan. Add the quinoa, lower the heat to a simmer, cover the pot, and cook for 15 to 20 minutes, or until the liquid is absorbed and the quinoa is soft.

3. Combine the cooked quinoa, feta cheese, Kalamata olives, cherry tomatoes, red onion, bell pepper, and parsley in a large bowl.

4. In a small bowl, whisk together the lemon juice, olive oil, salt, and pepper. Pour the dressing over the salad and toss to coat evenly.

Nutritional Information per Serving:

Kcal	Carbs	Protein	Fat	Sugar	Fiber
302	35g	8g	14g	4g	5g

Caprese Skewers

 10'   4

Ingredients:

16 small fresh mozzarella balls	1 tablespoon balsamic glaze
16 cherry tomatoes	Salt and pepper to taste
16 fresh basil leaves	Wooden skewers
2 tablespoons extra-virgin olive oil	

1. Thread a mozzarella ball, a fresh basil leaf, and a cherry tomato onto a wooden skewer. Continue until all ingredients have been utilized.

2. Position the skewers on a plate for serving.

3. Drizzle balsamic glaze and olive oil on the skewers.

4. Season with salt and pepper to taste5. Serve immediately and enjoy!

Nutritional Information (per serving):

Kcal	Carbs	Protein	Fat	Sugar	Fiber
1350	18.	122g	86g	8g	1g

Simple Vegetable Side Dishes

In this sub-chapter, we explore a collection of simple and flavorful vegetable side dishes that perfectly complement any meal. These dishes highlight the natural flavors of Mediterranean vegetables while keeping the preparation process quick and effortless. Whether you're looking for a light and refreshing side or a hearty accompaniment, these recipes will add a burst of color and nutrition to your table.

Garlic and Herb Sautéed Green Beans

 15'   2

Ingredients:

1 pound fresh green beans, trimmed	1 teaspoon dried thyme
2 tablespoons olive oil	Salt and pepper to taste
3 cloves garlic, minced	

1. In a large pan over medium heat, warm the olive oil.

2. Stir in the minced garlic, cooking it for a couple of minutes until fragrant.

3. Add the green beans and stir them in the oil and garlic in the skillet.

4. Season the green beans with salt, pepper, and dry thyme.

5. Sauté the green beans for 8 to 10 minutes with occasional turning, or until they are crisp and tender.

Nutritional Information (per serving):

Kcal	Carbs	Protein	Fat	Sugar	Fiber
103	9g	2g	7g	3g	3g

Lemon-Roasted Asparagus

 15' 2

Ingredients:

1 bunch asparagus, trimmed
2 tablespoons olive oil
Zest of 1 lemon
Juice of 1 lemon
Salt and pepper to taste

1. Preheat the oven to 425°F (220°C).

2. Place the trimmed asparagus spears on a baking sheet.

3. Drizzle olive oil over the asparagus and toss to coat evenly. Sprinkle lemon zest, lemon juice, salt, and pepper over the asparagus.

4. Roast in the preheated oven for 10-12 minutes, or until the asparagus is tender and slightly charred.

Nutritional Information (per serving):

Kcal	Carbs	Protein	Fat	Sugar	Fiber
80	3g	1g	7g	1g	1g

Grilled Eggplant with Herbed Yogurt Sauce

 20' 2

Ingredients:

2 medium eggplants, sliced into rounds
2 tablespoons olive oil
Salt and pepper to taste
1 cup plain Greek yogurt
1 tablespoon chopped fresh herbs (such as basil, parsley, or mint)
1 clove garlic, minced
1 tablespoon lemon juice

1. Turn on medium-high heat and prepare a grill or grill pan.

2. Sprinkle salt and pepper over the eggplant slices after brushing them with olive oil.

3. Grill the slices of eggplant for 3 to 4 minutes on each side, or until they are soft and have grill marks.

4. Meanwhile, in a small bowl, combine the Greek yogurt, chopped herbs, minced garlic, and lemon juice. Stir well to combine. Remove the grilled eggplant from the heat and arrange it on a serving platter.

6. Drizzle the herbed yogurt sauce over the grilled eggplant slices. Serve immediately as a delicious and satisfying vegetable side dish.

Nutritional Information (per serving):

Kcal	Carbs	Protein	Fat	Sugar	Fiber
181	16g	7g	10g	10g	6g

Wholesome Grain and Legume Salads

This section examines some healthful grain and legume salads that are not only tasty but also nutrient-dense. These salads are a great way to include whole grains and legumes in your diet while still enjoying the tastes and textures of items with a Mediterranean influence.

Steamed Broccoli with Lemon and Parmesan	Tomato and Mozzarella Salad with Cannellini Beans

 10' 2   15' 2

Ingredients:

1 pound broccoli florets	2 tablespoons grated Parmesan cheese
2 tablespoons olive oil	Salt and pepper to taste
Zest of 1 lemon	
Juice of 1 lemon	

1. Turn on medium-high heat and prepare a grill or grill pan.

2. Sprinkle salt and pepper over the eggplant slices after brushing them with olive oil.

3. Grill the slices of eggplant for 3 to 4 minutes on each side, or until they are soft and have grill marks.

5. Drizzle olive oil over the broccoli and sprinkle lemon zest, lemon juice, grated Parmesan cheese, salt, and pepper.

6. Toss the broccoli gently to coat it with the flavors.

7. Serve hot as a nutritious and satisfying side dish.

Nutritional Information (per serving):

Kcal	Carbs	Protein	Fat	Sugar	Fiber
114	8g	4g	8g	2g	3g

Ingredients:

2 cups cherry tomatoes, halved	2 tablespoons balsamic vinegar
1 cup cannellini beans, drained and rinsed	2 tablespoons extra-virgin olive oil
8 ounces fresh mozzarella cheese, diced	Salt and pepper to taste
¼ cup chopped fresh basil	

1. In a large mixing bowl, combine the cherry tomatoes, cannellini beans, diced mozzarella cheese, and chopped basil.

2. Combine the balsamic vinegar, olive oil, salt, and pepper in a small bowl.

3. Pour the dressing over the salad of tomatoes and mozzarella and gently toss to combine.

4. To enable the flavors to mingle, either serve the salad right away or marinate it for 30 minutes in the fridge.

Nutritional Information (per serving):

Kcal	Carbs	Protein	Fat	Sugar	Fiber
295	11g	16g	20g	4g	5g

Lentil Salad with Feta and Mint

 25' 2

Ingredients

1 cup green lentils
3 cups water
½ cup crumbled feta cheese
¼ cup chopped fresh mint leaves

¼ cup diced red onion
2 tablespoons lemon juice
2 tablespoons extra-virgin olive oil
Salt and pepper to taste

1. Drain the lentils after giving them a cold water rinse.

2. Bring the water to a boil in a saucepan. Low-heat the lentils after adding them.

3. Place the lentils in a covered pot and boil for 20 to 25 minutes, or until they are soft but still maintain their form.

4. Let the cooked lentils cool after draining them.

5. Combine the cooked lentils, feta cheese crumbles, chopped mint leaves, and red onion cubes in a large mixing dish.

6. Combine the lemon juice, olive oil, salt, and pepper in a small bowl.

7. After adding the dressing, incorporate the lentil mixture by gently tossing.

8. Serve the lentil salad with feta and mint chilled or at room temperature.

Nutritional Information (per serving):

Kcal	Carbs	Protein	Fat	Sugar	Fiber
282	29g	16g	12g	2g	14g

Quick Pickles and Fermented Veggies

In this sub-chapter, we explore the art of pickling and fermentation, offering a variety of quick and easy recipes to enhance your Mediterranean-inspired meals. From crispy pickles to probiotic-rich sauerkraut, these recipes will elevate your salads and sides.

Quick Pickled Cucumbers

 15' 2

Ingredients:

2 medium cucumbers, thinly sliced
½ cup white vinegar
¼ cup water
2 tablespoons sugar
1 tablespoon salt

1 teaspoon mustard seeds
½ teaspoon dill seeds
½ teaspoon black peppercorns
2 cloves garlic, crushed

1. In a small saucepan, combine the white vinegar, water, sugar, salt, mustard seeds, dill seeds, black peppercorns, and crushed garlic.

2. Over medium heat, bring the liquid to a boil while stirring until the salt and sugar have dissolved.

3. Turn off the heat and let the pickling liquid gently cool.

4. Put the cucumber slices in a jar or other container. Make sure the cucumbers are well immersed in the pickling liquid before pouring it over them.

5. At least an hour before serving, allow the cucumbers to marinate in the pickling juice.

Nutritional Information (per serving):

Kcal	Carbs	Protein	Fat	Sugar	Fiber
53	11g	1g	1g	8g	1g

Lacto-Fermented Sauerkraut

 30' + fermentation time   *2*

Ingredients:

1 small head green cabbage	1 teaspoon caraway seeds (optional)
1 tablespoon sea salt	

1. Remove the outer leaves of the cabbage and set them aside. Thinly slice the cabbage, discarding the core.

2. In a large mixing bowl, combine the sliced cabbage, sea salt, and caraway seeds (if using).

3. Massage and squeeze the cabbage with your hands for about 10 minutes until it starts releasing its juices.

4. Pack the cabbage tightly into a clean glass jar, pressing it down with a spoon or your hands to ensure it is submerged in its own juices.

5. Place one of the reserved cabbage leaves on top of the packed cabbage to help keep it submerged.

6. Cover the jar with a clean cloth or paper towel and secure it with a rubber band.

7. Let the jar sit at room temperature for 3-10 days, depending on your desired level of fermentation. Check the sauerkraut daily, pressing it down to keep it submerged.

8. Once the sauerkraut reaches your preferred level of tanginess, transfer the jar to the refrigerator to slow down the fermentation process.

Nutritional Information (per serving):

Kcal	Carbs	Protein	Fat	Sugar	Fiber
44	10g	2g	0g	5g	5g

Mediterranean Style Pickled Vegetables

 20'   *2*

Ingredients:

1 cup sliced cucumbers	½ cups of water
1 cup sliced bell peppers (assorted colors)	1 tablespoon sugar
	1 tablespoon salt
	1 teaspoon dried oregano
1 cup sliced red onion	1 teaspoon dried basil
1 cup sliced carrots	½ teaspoon red pepper flakes
½ cup white vinegar	

1. In a medium saucepan, combine the white vinegar, water, sugar, salt, dried oregano, dried basil, and red pepper flakes.

2. Bring the mixture to a boil over medium heat, stirring until the sugar and salt have dissolved.

3. Remove the saucepan from the heat and let the pickling liquid cool slightly.

4. Place the sliced cucumbers, bell peppers, red onion, and carrots in a jar or container.

5. Pour the pickling liquid over the vegetables, making sure they are completely submerged.

6. Let the vegetables marinate in the pickling liquid for at least 2 hours in the refrigerator before serving.

7. Serve the Mediterranean-style pickled vegetables as a refreshing and tangy side dish.

Nutritional Information (per serving):

Kcal	Carbs	Protein	Fat	Sugar	Fiber
59	12g	1g	0g	8g	2g

Spicy Carrot and Jalapeno Pickles

 15' 2

Ingredients:

2 cups sliced carrots
2 jalapeno peppers, sliced
2 cloves garlic, minced
1 cup white vinegar
1 cup water

2 tablespoons sugar
1 tablespoon salt
1 teaspoon black peppercorns
½ teaspoon crushed red pepper flakes

1. In a medium saucepan, combine the white vinegar, water, sugar, salt, black peppercorns, and crushed red pepper flakes.

2. Over medium heat, bring the liquid to a boil while stirring until the salt and sugar have dissolved.

3. Turn off the heat and let the pickling liquid gently cool.

4. Arrange the jalapeño peppers, minced garlic, and carrot slices in a jar or other container.

5. Cover the veggies fully with the pickling liquid by pouring it over them.

6. To enable the flavors to meld, let the pickles marinate in the fridge for at least 4 hours before serving.

7. Serve the spicy carrot and jalapeno pickles as a zesty and crunchy condiment.

Nutritional Information (per serving):

Kcal	Carbs	Protein	Fat	Sugar	Fiber
68	14g	1g	0g	9g	2g

CHAPTER 5: *Fast and Flavorful Main Courses*

We'll look at a range of quick and delectable main dishes in this chapter that are ideal for people who are on the go and eating a Mediterranean diet. You can quickly make delicious dinners with these dishes' vivid flavors and healthy ingredients. You may choose from a variety of cuisines to suit your preferences and dietary requirements, including one-pot pasta recipes, seafood specialties, and vegetarian selections. Let's dig in and learn about these scrumptious and quick main dishes with a Mediterranean influence!

You'll be taken on a gourmet tour of many quick-to-prepare and flavor-packed main dish alternatives in Chapter 5. You can maintain a well-balanced Mediterranean diet while saving time in the kitchen with the aid of these dishes. To accommodate a range of dietary requirements and taste preferences, each area will have a distinctive collection of dishes.

One-Pot Pasta and Grain Recipes

We'll look at delectable one-pot pasta and grain recipes in this section that perfectly encapsulate the tastes of the Mediterranean. These dishes are ideal for people who are busy and want to eat well without spending a lot of time in the kitchen. Each dish uses healthy components as well as bright herbs and spices to produce a mouthwatering result.

Mediterranean Baked Salmon

 20' 2

Ingredients:

4 salmon fillets (50g)	Salt and pepper to taste
2 tablespoons olive oil	1 cup cherry tomatoes, halved
2 tablespoons lemon juice	1/4 cup Kalamata olives, pitted and halved
2 cloves garlic, minced	2 tablespoons chopped fresh parsley, for garnish
1 teaspoon dried oregano	Lemon wedges, for serving
1/2 teaspoon dried basil	
1/2 teaspoon dried thyme	

1. Set the oven to 360°F (180°C) before using. Use parchment paper to line a baking sheet or gently oil it.

2. On the prepared baking sheet, arrange the salmon fillets.

3. Combine the olive oil, lemon juice, chopped garlic, dried oregano, dried basil, dried thyme, salt, and pepper in a small dish.

4. Make sure the salmon fillets are uniformly covered before drizzling the mixture over them.

5. Scatter the halved cherry tomatoes and Kalamata olives around the salmon on the baking sheet.

6. Bake in the preheated oven for about 15 minutes, or until the salmon is cooked through and flakes easily with a fork.

7. Remove the baking sheet from the oven and let the salmon rest for a few minutes.

8. Garnish with chopped fresh parsley, and serve with lemon wedges on the side.

Nutritional Information (per serving):

Kcal	Carbs	Protein	Fat	Sugar	Fiber
326	3g	24g	23g	1g	1g

Quick Seafood and Fish Dishes

In this sub-chapter, we dive into the world of quick and delightful seafood and fish dishes that are perfect for incorporating the flavors of the Mediterranean into your diet. From succulent shrimp and tender salmon fillets to deliciously grilled squid and zesty fish tacos, these recipes showcase the versatility and health benefits of seafood. These meals will take you to the Mediterranean shore thanks to their vivid colors and fresh ingredients. These fast and simple dishes will definitely sate your desires while giving you a wholesome and delectable eating experience, whether you adore seafood or are trying to include more marine delicacies in your meals.

Note: Cooking times may vary depending on the thickness of the seafood or fish, so adjust accordingly and ensure they are cooked through before serving.

Grilled Lemon Herb Salmon

 10'   10'   2

Ingredients:

4 salmon fillets (about 2/3 ounces each)
2 tablespoons olive oil
2 cloves garlic, minced
Zest and juice of 1 lemon
1 tablespoon chopped fresh dill
Salt and pepper to taste

5. Take the salmon off the grill and give it a moment to rest before serving.

6. Add a squeeze of fresh lemon juice to the salmon before serving

Nutritional Information (per serving):

Kcal	Carbs	Protein	Fat	Sugar	Fiber
150	1g	8g	12g	0g	0g

1. To create the marinade, combine the olive oil, minced garlic, lemon juice, lemon zest, finely chopped fresh dill, salt, and pepper in a small bowl.

2. Spoon the marinade over the salmon fillets that have been placed in a shallow dish. Ensure that the fillets are well coated. Give the fish 10 minutes to marinate.

3. Set the grill's temperature to medium-high.

4. Grill the salmon fillets skin-side down after marinating. Grill the salmon for 4–5 minutes on each side, or until it reaches the desired doneness.

Garlic Butter Shrimp Pasta

 10' 15' 2

Ingredients:

6 ounces linguine or spaghetti
10/12 ounces large shrimp, peeled and deveined
4 tablespoons unsalted butter
4 cloves garlic, minced

1/4 teaspoon red pepper flakes (optional)
Juice of 1 lemon
Salt and pepper to taste
Chopped fresh parsley for garnish

1. Light the fire underneath the pot, then wait for the water to boil. Pasta or spaghetti should be salted and cooked per the directions on the box until al dente.

2. During the pasta cooking process, Melt the butter in a large pan over medium heat. When aromatic, add the minced garlic and red pepper flakes (if using) and cook for approximately a minute.

3. Add the shrimp to the skillet and cook them for two to three minutes on each side, or until they are opaque and pink.

4. Add the pasta al dente to the skillet and toss it with the shrimp, garlic butter, and lemon juice. Season with salt and pepper to taste.

5. Cook for an additional 1-2 minutes, allowing the flavors to combine.

6. Remove from heat and garnish with chopped fresh parsley.

Nutritional Information (per serving):

Kcal	Carbs	Protein	Fat	Sugar	Fiber
412	44g	30g	12g	1g	2g

Satisfying Poultry and Meat Recipes

This sub-chapter offers a variety of Mediterranean-inspired meat and poultry recipes that are flavorful and satisfying. These meals, which feature grilled chicken, succulent turkey cutlets, and flavorful lamb kofta kebabs, reflect the vibrant flavors of the Mediterranean region. Each meal is carefully crafted to highlight the natural tastes of the ingredients and provide a filling and nutritious evening.

Note: Cooking times may vary depending on the thickness of the poultry or meat, so adjust accordingly and ensure they are cooked through before serving.

Note: Internal temperature:

- internal temperature of chicken 165°F (74°C)
- **minimum** internal temperature of pork 150°F (65°C)
- internal temperature of turkey 160°F (70/72°C)
- For beef, approximate temperatures are 120°F (48-50°C for rare), 125°F (51-53°C for medium rare), 130°F (54-57°C for medium) and 145°F (63°C or higher for well-done)

Herb-Roasted Chicken Breast with Lemon

 10' 25' 2

Ingredients:

4 chicken breasts, boneless and skinless
2 tablespoons olive oil
2 cloves garlic, minced
1 tablespoon fresh rosemary, chopped

1 tablespoon fresh thyme leaves
Juice and zest of 1 lemon
Salt and pepper to taste

1. Set the oven temperature to 425°F (220°C).

2. Arrange the chicken breasts on a parchment-lined baking pan.

3. Combine the lemon juice, lemon zest, rosemary, thyme, olive oil, minced garlic, salt, and pepper in a small bowl. Mix thoroughly.

4. Apply the herb mixture to the chicken breasts' top and bottom surfaces.

5. Roast the chicken in the preheated oven for 20 to 25 minutes, or until a meat thermometer inserted into the thickest portion of the chicken breast registers a temperature of 165°F (74°C).

6. Take the chicken out of the oven and let it rest before serving.

Nutritional Information (per serving):

Kcal	Carbs	Protein	Fat	Sugar	Fiber
309	1g	45g	12g	0.24g	0.4g

Grilled Balsamic Glazed Pork Chops

 10' 15' 30' 2

Ingredients:

4 pork chops, bone-in
1/4 cup balsamic
vinegar
2 tablespoons olive oil
2 tablespoons honey
2 cloves garlic,
minced

1 teaspoon Dijon
mustard
1 teaspoon dried
rosemary
Salt and pepper to
taste

1. In a small bowl, whisk together the balsamic vinegar, olive oil, honey, minced garlic, Dijon mustard, dried rosemary, salt, and pepper to make the marinade.

2. Place the pork chops in a shallow dish and pour the marinade over them, ensuring they are well coated. Cover the dish and marinate it in the refrigerator for at least 30 minutes.

3. Preheat the grill to medium-high heat.

4. Remove the pork chops from the marinade, reserving the marinade for basting.

5. Grill the pork chops for 6 minutes on each side, or until they reach an internal temperature of 160°F (70°C) when measured with a meat thermometer.

6. While grilling, baste the pork chops with the reserved marinade.

7. Remove the pork chops from the grill and let them rest for a few minutes before serving. Serve the grilled balsamic-glazed pork chops with your favorite side dishes.

Nutritional Information (per serving):

Kcal	Carbs	Protein	Fat	Sugar	Fiber
368	12g	31g	20g	11g	0.3g

Mediterranean Style Beef Kebabs

 15' 15' 1h 2

Ingredients:

1 pound beef sirloin,
cut into 1-inch cubes
1 red bell pepper, cut
into 1-inch pieces
1 green bell pepper,
cut into 1-inch pieces
1 red onion, cut into 1-
inch pieces
8 cherry tomatoes

2 tablespoons olive oil
2 cloves garlic,
minced
1 tablespoon lemon
juice
1 teaspoon dried
oregano
1 teaspoon dried
thyme
Salt and pepper to
taste

1. In a bowl, combine the olive oil, minced garlic, lemon juice, dried oregano, dried thyme, salt, and pepper to make the marinade.

2. Place the beef cubes in a shallow dish, and pour the marinade over them. Toss to coat the beef evenly. Cover the dish and marinate in the refrigerator for at least 1 hour.

3. Preheat the grill to medium-high heat.

4. Thread the marinated beef cubes onto skewers, alternating with the bell peppers, onions, and cherry tomatoes.

5. Grill the kebabs for 4-6 minutes per side, or until the beef reaches your desired level of doneness.

6. Remove the kebabs from the grill and let them rest for a few minutes before serving. Serve with a side of tzatziki sauce or your favorite dipping sauce.

Nutritional Information (per serving):

Kcal	Carbs	Protein	Fat	Sugar	Fiber

321	6g	24g	22g	3g	2g

Herb-Marinated Grilled Turkey Cutlets

 15' 10' 1h 2

Ingredients:

4 turkey cutlets
2 tablespoons olive oil
2 cloves garlic, minced
Salt and pepper to taste

2 tablespoons chopped fresh herbs (such as rosemary, thyme, and parsley)
Juice of 1 lemon

1. To create the marinade, combine the olive oil, minced garlic, finely chopped fresh herbs, lemon juice, salt, and pepper in a bowl.

2. Spread the marinade over the turkey cutlets in a shallow dish. Ensure that the cutlets are well covered. For at least an hour, marinate the meal in the fridge with a cover on.

3. Set the grill's temperature to medium-high.

4. Take the turkey cutlets out of the marinade and throw away any leftover marinade.

5. Use a meat thermometer to check that the turkey cutlets' internal temperature is 165°F (74°C), or grill them for 4 minutes on each side.

6. Take the turkey cutlets from the grill and give them a moment to rest before serving.

7. Slice the turkey cutlets and serve with your choice of side dishes.

Nutritional Information (per serving):

Kcal	Carbs	Protein	Fat	Sugar	Fiber
240	1g	35g	10g	0.3g	0.3g

Flavorful Lamb Kofta Kebabs

 20' 15' ⊗ 2

Ingredients:

12 ounces ground lamb
1/2 onion, finely chopped
2 cloves garlic, minced
1 tablespoon chopped fresh parsley
1 tablespoon chopped fresh mint

1 teaspoon ground cumin
1 teaspoon ground coriander
1/2 teaspoon ground cinnamon
Salt and pepper to taste

1. In a large bowl, combine the ground lamb, finely chopped onion, minced garlic, chopped fresh parsley, chopped fresh mint, ground cumin, ground coriander, ground cinnamon, salt, and pepper. Mix well until all the ingredients are evenly incorporated.

2. Split the lamb mixture into 8 equal bits, and then give each one the shape of a kebab.

3. Set the grill's temperature to medium-high.

4. Grill the lamb kofta kebabs on each side for 4-6 minutes, or until they are well heated through and have a light char.

5. Take the kebabs off the grill and give them time to rest before serving.

6. Put some tzatziki sauce or your preferred dipping sauce on the side and serve the tasty lamb kofta kebabs.

Nutritional Information (per serving):

Kcal	Carbs	Protein	Fat	Sugar	Fiber
332	2g	19g	26g	0.56g	0.7g

Grilled Honey Mustard Chicken

 10' 10' 30' 2

Ingredients:

4 boneless, skinless chicken breasts
1/4 cup Dijon mustard
2 tablespoons honey
2 tablespoons olive oil
2 cloves garlic, minced
1 teaspoon dried thyme
Salt and pepper to taste
Chopped fresh parsley for garnish

1. To create the marinade, combine the honey, Dijon mustard, olive oil, chopped garlic, dried thyme, salt, and pepper in a bowl.

2. Pour the marinade over the chicken breasts that you've placed in a shallow dish. Assure a thorough coating of the chicken. In the refrigerator, let them marinate for about 30 minutes.

3. Set the grill's temperature to medium-high.

4. Take the marinade off the chicken breasts and throw it away.

5. Grill the chicken breasts for 5 to 6 minutes on each side, or until they are well cooked and register 165 degrees Fahrenheit (74 degrees Celsius).

6. Take the chicken off the grill and give it a moment to rest. Add freshly cut parsley as a garnish.

7. Serve with a side of salad or roasted vegetables.

Nutritional Information (per serving):

Kcal	Carbs	Protein	Fat	Sugar	Fiber
347	10g	45g	12g	8g	1g

Flavorful Vegetarian and Vegan Meals

This sub-chapter's recipes emphasize the use of healthful foods such vegetables, legumes, grains, herbs, and spices, all of which add to the dishes' rich tastes and health advantages. Each meal blends the particular tastes of the Mediterranean area, whether it be stuffed bell peppers, Greek chickpea salad, Caprese-stuffed Portobello mushrooms, or ratatouille.

These delectable vegetarian and vegan dishes offer a mix of necessary nutrients in addition to being delicious. They are a nutrient-dense alternative for anyone looking to increase the number of plant-based foods in their diet since they are high in fiber, plant-based proteins, vitamins, and minerals.

Vegetable Stir-Fry with Tofu

 15'   10'   2

Ingredients:

1 block firm tofu, drained and cubed
2 tablespoons soy sauce
1 tablespoon sesame oil
2 tablespoons vegetable oil
2 cloves garlic, minced
1 tablespoon grated ginger
1 red bell pepper, thinly sliced
1 yellow bell pepper, thinly sliced
1 small zucchini, sliced
1 cup broccoli florets
1 cup snap peas
2 tablespoons hoisin sauce
1 tablespoon rice vinegar
Salt and pepper to taste
Chopped green onions for garnish
Cooked rice or noodles for serving

1. Combine the cubed tofu, sesame oil, and soy sauce in a bowl. To coat the tofu, gently toss. Give it some time to marinate.

2. In a large skillet or wok, heat the vegetable oil over medium-high heat.

3. Stir-fry the grated ginger and minced garlic in the heated oil for approximately 30 seconds, or until fragrant.

4. Add the tofu that has been marinated to the skillet and cook, turning regularly, for 3 to 4 minutes, or until the tofu is golden brown.

5. Fill the skillet with the sliced bell peppers, zucchini, broccoli florets, and snap peas. Stir-fry the veggies for a further 4-5 minutes, or until they are crisp-tender.

6. In a small bowl, whisk together the hoisin sauce and rice vinegar. Pour the sauce over the stir-fried vegetables and tofu. Stir well to coat everything evenly. Season with salt and pepper to taste.

7.Remove from the heat and garnish with chopped green onions. Serve with tofu over cooked rice or noodles.

Nutritional Information (per serving):

Kcal	Carbs	Protein	Fat	Sugar	Fiber
170	11g	5g	11g	5g	2g

Lentil and Vegetable Curry

 15'   25'   2

Ingredients:

1 cup dried red lentils, rinsed

2 tablespoons vegetable oil

1 medium onion, chopped

2 cloves garlic, minced

1 tablespoon grated ginger

2 teaspoons curry powder

1 teaspoon ground cumin

1/2 teaspoon ground turmeric

1/4 teaspoon cayenne pepper (optional, for heat)

1 can (7 ounces) coconut milk

1 can (10 ounces) diced tomatoes

2 cups chopped vegetables (such as bell peppers, carrots, and peas)

Salt and pepper

Fresh cilantro

Cooked rice or naan bread for serving

1. Bring 3 cups of water to a boil in a big saucepan. Cook the rinsed lentils for a further ten to fifteen minutes, or until they are soft. Drain, then set apart.

2. Set the vegetable oil in the same saucepan over medium heat. Cook the chopped onion for 5 minutes, or until it softens.

3. Include the curry powder, cumin, turmeric, cayenne pepper (if using), chopped garlic, grated ginger, and grated ginger. Cook for 1 minute, stirring often, until aromatic.

4. Add the chopped tomatoes with their juices and the coconut milk. To blend, stir. To the saucepan, add the cooked lentils and the chopped veggies. To taste, add salt and pepper to the food.

5. Bring the mixture to a simmer and let it cook for 10 minutes, stirring occasionally, until the vegetables are tender.

Nutritional Information (per serving):

Kcal	Carbs	Protein	Fat	Sugar	Fiber
483	45g	16g	29g	5g	7g

Mediterranean Stuffed Bell Peppers

 15'   40' 2

Ingredients:

3 bell peppers (any color), tops removed and seeds removed

1 cup cooked quinoa

1 can (10 ounces) chickpeas, rinsed and drained

1/2 cup diced tomatoes

1/2 cup chopped Kalamata olives

1/4 cup crumbled feta cheese (optional for vegans)

2 tablespoons chopped fresh parsley

1 tablespoon lemon juice

1 tablespoon olive oil

2 cloves garlic, minced

1 teaspoon dried oregano

Salt and pepper to taste

1. Preheat the oven to 375°F (190°C).

2. Place the bell peppers in a baking dish, standing upright.

3. In a large bowl, combine the cooked quinoa, chickpeas, diced tomatoes, Kalamata olives, feta cheese (if using), parsley, lemon juice, olive oil, minced garlic, dried oregano, salt, and pepper. Mix well.

4. Spoon the quinoa mixture into the bell peppers, filling them to the top. Cover the baking dish with foil and bake for 30 minutes.

6. Remove the foil and bake for an additional 10 minutes until the bell peppers are tender and slightly charred. Remove them from the oven and let them cool for a few minutes before serving.

Nutritional Information (per serving):

Kcal	Carbs	Protein	Fat	Sugar	Fiber
285	33g	9g	13g	7g	8g

Greek Chickpea Salad

 15 min 2

Ingredients:

1 can (10 ounces) chickpeas, rinsed and drained
1 English cucumber, diced
1 cup cherry tomatoes, halved
1/2 cup diced red onion
1/2 cup diced Kalamata olives

1/2 cup crumbled feta cheese (optional for vegans)
2 tablespoons chopped fresh parsley
2 tablespoons lemon juice
2 tablespoons extra-virgin olive oil
1 teaspoon dried oregano
Salt and pepper to taste

1. In a large bowl, combine the chickpeas, diced cucumber, cherry tomatoes, red onion, Kalamata olives, crumbled feta cheese (if using), chopped parsley, lemon juice, olive oil, dried oregano, salt, and pepper.

2. Toss well to combine and coat everything in the dressing. Adjust the seasoning if needed.

4. Let the salad sit for at least 10 minutes to allow the flavors to meld together. Serve the Greek chickpea salad chilled or at room temperature.

Nutritional Information (per serving):

Kcal	Carbs	Protein	Fat	Sugar	Fiber
364	36g	12g	19g	8g	10g

Caprese Stuffed Portobello Mushrooms

 15' 20' 2

Ingredients:

4 large Portobello mushrooms, stems removed
4 slices fresh mozzarella cheese (or vegan mozzarella alternative)
4 slices ripe tomato

Fresh basil leaves
2 tablespoons balsamic glaze
2 tablespoons extra-virgin olive oil
Salt and pepper to taste

1. Set the oven temperature to 375°F (190°C).

2. Arrange the Portobello mushrooms with their gills facing up on a baking pan.

3. Add salt and pepper to each mushroom and drizzle olive oil over them.

4. For 15 minutes, roast the mushrooms in the preheated oven.

5. After taking the mushrooms out of the oven, garnish each one with a piece of mozzarella cheese, a tomato slice, and some fresh basil.

6. Bake the mushrooms once more in the oven for 5 more minutes, or until the cheese is melted and bubbling.

7. Drizzle the balsamic glaze over the stuffed mushrooms.

Nutritional Information (per serving):

Kcal	Carbs	Protein	Fat	Sugar	Fiber
172	7g	8g	13g	5g	1g

CHAPTER 6: *Express Soups and Stews*

The world of fast and nourishing soups and stews, influenced by the Mediterranean culinary heritage, is explored in Chapter 6. These dishes combine substantial foods, fragrant herbs, and delicious spices to create a bowl of comfort and sustenance. This chapter offers both light soups and heavy stews, so you're covered. Let's investigate the mouthwatering flavors of Mediterranean stews and soups!

Hearty Vegetable Soups

This chapter's sub-chapter examines a variety of filling and healthful vegetable soup recipes. These soups are rich and warming because they are loaded with a variety of vegetables, herbs, and spices.

These recipes highlight the flexibility of vegetables and their capacity to produce filling and delectable soups, from the traditional Minestrone Soup rich with vegetables and beans to the creamy and velvety Roasted Butternut Squash Soup. The dishes are designed to be simple to make, so you can sit down to a filling supper quickly.

Tuscan White Bean Soup

 10'   25'   2

Ingredients:

1/2 can of white beans, drained and rinsed
1 onion, chopped
3 garlic cloves, minced
2 carrots, diced
2 celery stalks, diced
4 cups vegetable broth
1 can diced tomatoes
1 teaspoon dried rosemary
1 teaspoon dried thyme
Salt and pepper to taste
Fresh parsley for garnish

1. Sauté the onion and garlic in a big saucepan until they are transparent.

2. Include the celery and carrots in the saucepan and simmer for a few minutes, until they're just beginning to soften.

3. Fill the saucepan with the chopped tomatoes, vegetable broth, dry rosemary, and dried thyme.

4. After the mixture comes to a boil, lower the heat and let it simmer for around 20 minutes.

5. To taste, add salt and pepper to the food. Hot soup should be served with fresh parsley on top.

Nutritional Information (per serving):

Kcal	Carbs	Protein	Fat	Sugar	Fiber
621	114g	41g	2g	7g	27g

Minestrone Soup

 15' 25' 2

Ingredients:

1 onion, chopped
2 carrots, diced
2 celery stalks, diced
3 garlic cloves, minced
1 zucchini, diced
1 cup diced tomatoes
4 cups vegetable broth

1 can kidney beans, drained and rinsed
1 cup small pasta (such as ditalini or elbow macaroni)
1 teaspoon dried basil
1 teaspoon dried oregano
Salt and pepper to taste
Fresh basil for garnish

1. Soften the onion, carrots, celery, and garlic in a big saucepan.

2. Fill the saucepan with the kidney beans, zucchini, diced tomatoes, vegetable broth, dried basil, and dried oregano.

3. After bringing the mixture to a boil, lower the heat and let it simmer for around 15 minutes.

4. Add the pasta to the saucepan and boil it until al dente, as directed on the packet.

5. To taste, add salt and pepper to the food.

6. Ladle the heated soup into bowls and top with fresh basil.

Nutritional Information (per serving):

Kcal	Carbs	Protein	Fat	Sugar	Fiber
199	38g	8g	1g	6g	5g

Moroccan Spiced Lentil Soup

 10' 30' 2

Ingredients

1 cup dried red lentils
1 onion, chopped
2 carrots, diced
2 celery stalks, diced
3 garlic cloves, minced
1 can diced tomatoes
Fresh cilantro for garnish
Salt and pepper

4 cups vegetable broth
1 teaspoon ground cumin
1 teaspoon ground coriander
1/2 teaspoon ground turmeric

:

1. Red lentils should be rinsed in cold water and kept aside after.

2. Soften the onion, carrots, celery, and garlic in a big saucepan.

3. Fill the saucepan with the lentils, diced tomatoes, vegetable broth, cumin, coriander, and turmeric. 4. After the mixture comes to a boil, lower the heat and simmer the mixture for about 20 minutes, or until the lentils are cooked through.

5. To taste, add salt and pepper to the food.

6. Ladle the heated soup into bowls and top with fresh cilantro.

Nutritional Information (per serving):

Kcal	Carbs	Protein	Fat	Sugar	Fiber
231	43g	14g	1g	4g	7g

Roasted Butternut Squash Soup

 15' 45' 2

Ingredients:

1 large butternut squash, peeled, seeded, and cut into cubes
1 onion, chopped
3 cloves of garlic, minced
2 carrots, peeled and chopped
2 celery stalks, chopped
4 cups vegetable broth
1 teaspoon dried thyme
1/2 teaspoon ground cinnamon
1/4 teaspoon ground nutmeg
Salt and pepper to taste
2 tablespoons olive oil
Optional toppings: roasted pumpkin seeds, fresh herbs, or a drizzle of cream

1. Set the oven's temperature to 425°F (220°C). Use parchment paper to cover a baking sheet.

2. Arrange the cubes of butternut squash on the baking sheet that has been prepared and drizzle with 1 tablespoon of olive oil. Toss to evenly coat the squash.

3. Roast the butternut squash for 30-35 minutes, or until it is soft and caramelized, in the preheated oven. Place aside.

4. Heat the final tablespoon of olive oil in a big soup pot over medium heat. Add the celery, carrots, onion, and garlic. The veggies should be sautéed for about 5 minutes, or until they are soft.

5. Add the vegetable broth, dried thyme, cinnamon, nutmeg, salt, and pepper to the saucepan along with the roasted butternut squash. To blend, stir.

6. After bringing the mixture to a boil, lower the heat and let it simmer for 15 to 20 minutes to let the flavors mingle.

7. Puree the soup in a normal or immersion blender until it is silky and creamy. When combining hot liquids, use caution.

8. Put the soup back in the pot and taste to see if the seasoning needs changing. To get the required consistency, add extra water or vegetable broth if the soup is too thick.

9. Reheat the soup over low heat if necessary.

10. Ladle the roasted butternut squash soup into bowls and garnish with your preferred toppings, such as roasted pumpkin seeds, fresh herbs, or a drizzle of cream.

Nutritional Information (per serving):

Kcal	Carbs	Protein	Fat	Sugar	Fiber
226	38g	4g	8g	9g	7g

Quick Seafood Stews

Mediterranean Fish Stew

 20' 2

Ingredients:

1 tablespoon olive oil
1 onion, chopped
2 garlic cloves, minced
1 red bell pepper, diced
1 yellow bell pepper, diced
1 can (10 ounces) diced tomatoes
1 cup vegetable broth
1 teaspoon oregano
1/2 teaspoon dried basil

1/2 teaspoon paprika
Salt and pepper to taste
10 ounces white fish fillets (such as cod or haddock), cut into chunks
1/2 cup pitted Kalamata olives
2 tablespoons chopped fresh parsley
Lemon for serving

1. Heat the olive oil in a big saucepan or Dutch oven over medium heat. Add the minced garlic and diced onion, and cook until aromatic and soft.

2. Stir in the diced red and yellow bell peppers and simmer for a few minutes, or until they begin to soften.

3. Add the veggie broth and diced tomatoes. Add the paprika, salt, pepper, dried basil, oregano, and basil leaves. Simmer the mixture for a little while.

4. Gently add the Kalamata olives and fish pieces to the stew. For approximately 10 minutes, or until the fish is cooked through and flakes readily with a fork, simmer the dish with the lid on.

5. Remove the pot from the heat and stir in the chopped fresh parsley. Serve with lemon

Nutritional Information (per serving):

Kcal	Carbs	Protein	Fat	Sugar	Fiber
208	10g	23g	9g	2g	1g

Spicy Shrimp and Tomato Stew

 25' 2

Ingredients:

1 tablespoon olive oil
1 onion, finely chopped
2 garlic cloves, minced
1 red bell pepper, diced
1 can (10 ounces) diced tomatoes
1 cup vegetable broth
1 teaspoon smoked paprika

1/2 teaspoon cayenne pepper (adjust according to your spice preference)
Salt and pepper to taste
10 ounces shrimp, peeled and deveined
2 tablespoons chopped fresh parsley
Crusty bread, for serving

1. In a big saucepan or Dutch oven, heat the olive oil over medium heat. When the onion is transparent, add the minced garlic and the diced onion.

2. Include the red bell pepper in the saucepan and stir occasionally for a few minutes, or until it begins to soften.

3. Add the veggie broth and diced tomatoes. Add salt, pepper, cayenne pepper, and smoked paprika after stirring. Simmer the mixture for a little while.

4. Add the shrimp to the pot and cook for about 5-7 minutes, or until the shrimp is pink and cooked through.

5. Stir in the chopped fresh parsley and let the stew simmer for another 2-3 minutes.

6. Serve hot with crusty bread for dipping.

Nutritional Information (per serving):

Kcal	Carbs	Protein	Fat	Sugar	Fiber
171	8g	24g	4g	2g	1g

Tuscan Seafood Cioppino

 35' 2

Ingredients:

2 tablespoons olive oil

1 onion, chopped

2 garlic cloves, minced

1 fennel bulb, thinly sliced

1 red bell pepper, diced

1 can (10 ounces) diced tomatoes

1 cup vegetable broth

1/2 cup dry white wine

1 teaspoon dried basil

1 teaspoon dried oregano

1/2 teaspoon red pepper flakes (adjust according to your spice preference)

Salt and pepper to taste

10 ounces mixed seafood (such as shrimp, scallops, mussels, and clams)

2 tablespoons chopped fresh parsley

Crusty bread, for serving

1. In a big saucepan or Dutch oven, heat the olive oil over medium heat. When the onion is transparent, add the minced garlic and the diced onion.

2. Include the chopped red bell pepper and sliced fennel in the saucepan and simmer for a few minutes, or until they begin to soften.

3. Add the vegetable broth, white wine, and chopped tomatoes. Add the red pepper flakes, dried oregano, dry basil, salt, and pepper. Simmer the mixture for a little while.

4. Gently add the mixed seafood to the pot and simmer for about 10 minutes, or until the seafood is cooked through and the shells of the mussels and clams have opened.

5. Stir in the chopped fresh parsley and let the cioppino simmer for another 2-3 minutes.

Nutritional Information (per serving):

Kcal	Carbs	Protein	Fat	Sugar	Fiber
256	14g	23g	9g	4g	3g

Comforting Legume Soups

In this sub-chapter, we explore a collection of comforting legume soups that are not only delicious but also packed with nutritional benefits. Legumes, such as beans and lentils, are a great source of plant-based protein, fiber, and essential nutrients. These hearty soups will warm you up on chilly days and provide you with a satisfying and nourishing meal.

Lentil and Vegetable Soup	Creamy Italian Spinach and Bean Soup

 30' 2

 30' 2

Ingredients:

1 tablespoon olive oil
1 onion, diced
2 carrots, diced
2 celery stalks, diced
3 garlic cloves, minced
1 cup dried lentils rinsed and drained
4 cups vegetable broth

1 can (10 ounces) diced tomatoes
1 teaspoon ground cumin
1 teaspoon ground coriander
Salt and pepper to taste
Fresh parsley, chopped, for garnish

1. Heat the olive oil in a big saucepan or Dutch oven over medium heat. Then, for approximately 5 minutes, sauté the chopped celery, onion, and carrots until they begin to soften.

2. Stir in the minced garlic and cook for an additional minute.

3. Fill the saucepan with the lentils, vegetable broth, chopped tomatoes, cumin, coriander, salt, and pepper. To blend, thoroughly stir.

4. Bring the mixture to a boil before turning down the heat. The lentils should be soft after 20 to 25 minutes of simmering under cover.

5. Spoon the lentil and vegetable soup into dishes and top with fresh parsley that has been chopped.

Nutritional Information (per serving):

Kcal	Carbs	Protein	Fat	Sugar	Fiber
256	39g	15g	5g	6g	16g

Ingredients

1 tablespoon olive oil
1 red onion, chopped
1 stalk celery, chopped
1 clove garlic, minced
1 can (10 ounce) of great white northern beans, rinsed and drained
1 can (5 ounce) of chicken broth

1/4 teaspoon ground black pepper
1/8 teaspoon dried Greek seasoning
2 cups water
1 bunch fresh spinach, rinsed and thinly sliced
1 tablespoon lemon juice

1.First, heat the oil in a pan and cook the onion and celery on medium for about 7 minutes, or until tender.

2. Add garlic and allow it to cook for 30 seconds.

3. Add the beans, broth, pepper, thyme, and water. Bring to a boil and reduce to a simmer for 15 minutes.

4. Set aside the bean and vegetable mixture. Blend the remaining soup using a food processor or blender and pour it back into the pot. Add back the beans and vegetables.

6. Boil, add the spinach, and cook for one minute. Add the lemon juice, and serve.

Nutritional Information (per serving):

Kcal	Carbs	Protein	Fat	Sugar	Fiber
443	73g	29g	4g	4g	19g

Italian Lima Bean Soup

 30' 2

Ingredients

1 tablespoon olive oil
1 red onion, chopped
1 stalk celery,
chopped 1 clove
garlic,
minced 1 (10 ounce)
can of lima beans,
rinsed and drained
1 (5 ounce) can
vegetable broth

1/4 teaspoon ground
black pepper
1/8 teaspoon dried
Italian seasoning
2 cups water
1 bunch fresh spinach,
rinsed and thinly
sliced
1 tablespoon lemon
juice

1. First, heat the oil in a pan and cook the onion and celery on medium for about 7 minutes, or until tender.

2. Add garlic and allow it to cook for 30 seconds.

3. Add the beans, broth, pepper, thyme, and water.

4. Bring to a boil and reduce to a simmer for 15 minutes.

5. Set aside the bean and vegetable mixture.

6. Blend the remaining soup using a food processor or blender and pour it back into the pot.

7. Add back the beans and vegetables.

8. Boil, add the spinach, and cook for one minute. Add the lemon juice, sprinkle with cheese, and serve.

Nutritional Information (per serving):

Kcal	Carbs	Protein	Fat	Sugar	Fiber
451	77g	27g	4g	11g	23g

Moroccan Fava Bean Soup

 30' 2

Ingredients

2 tablespoons extra
virgin olive oil
1 large yellow onion,
chopped
4 cups water, or more
to taste
1 tablespoon all-
purpose flour
1 teaspoon corn-
starch salt
Ground black pepper
to taste
10 ounces - tomatoes,
diced
1 (10 ounce) can fava
beans, drained

1 bunch fresh cilantro,
chopped
1 bunch fresh parsley,
chopped
20 fresh mint leaves,
chopped
1 teaspoon ground
paprika
1 teaspoon ground
turmeric
1 teaspoon ground
ginger
1/2 teaspoon harissa
1 pinch saffron
threads
1/2 cup cherry
tomatoes, halved

1. First, heat the oil in a pot over medium heat.

2. Add the onion and allow it to cook until translucent.

3. Add all of the vegetable ingredients except the tomatoes.

4. Add water and cook over medium heat for 30 minutes.

5. Mix the soup liquid with flour and cornstarch and add it to the soup. Add the tomatoes and boil.

7. Simmer over low heat for ten minutes or until thickened. Add salt and pepper to taste.

Nutritional Information (per serving):

Kcal	Carbs	Protein	Fat	Sugar	Fiber
212	28g	8g	8g	22g	8g

Vegetarian Moroccan Fava Bean Soup

 30' 2

Ingredients

2 tablespoons canola oil

1 large red onion, chopped

4 cups water, or more to taste

1 tablespoon all-purpose flour

1 teaspoon cornstarch salt and ground black pepper to taste

10 ounces - tomatoes, diced

1 (10 ounce) can fava beans,

1 bunch fresh cilantro, chopped

1 bunch fresh parsley, chopped

20 fresh mint leaves, chopped

1 teaspoon ground paprika

1 teaspoon ground turmeric

1 teaspoon ground ginger

1/2 teaspoon harissa

1 pinch saffron threads

1/2 cup tomatillos or green tomatoes, halved

1. First, heat the oil in a pot over medium heat.

2. Add the onion and allow it to cook until translucent.

3. Add all of the vegetable ingredients except the tomatoes.

4. Add water and cook over medium heat for 30 minutes.

5. Mix the soup liquid with flour and cornstarch and add it to the soup. Add the tomatoes and boil. Simmer over low heat for ten minutes or until thickened.

Nutritional Information (per serving):

Kcal	Carbs	Protein	Fat	Sugar	Fiber
247	33g	12g	8g	32g	9g

Mediterranean Tomato&Chickpea Soup

 30'   2

Ingredients

2 tablespoons olive oil

1 large yellow onion, chopped

4 cups water, or more to taste

1 tablespoon all-purpose flour

1 teaspoon cornstarch salt and ground black pepper to taste

10 ounces tomatoes, diced

1 (10 ounce) can chickpeas, drained

1 bunch fresh cilantro, chopped

1 bunch fresh parsley, chopped

20 fresh mint leaves, chopped

1 teaspoon ground paprika

1 teaspoon ground turmeric

1 teaspoon ground ginger

1/2 teaspoon harissa

1 pinch saffron threads

1/2 cup small tomatoes, halved

Procedure

1. First, heat the oil in a pot over medium heat.

2. Add the onion and allow it to cook until translucent.

3. Add all of the vegetable ingredients except the tomatoes. Add water and cook over medium heat for 30 minutes.

4. Mix the soup liquid with flour and cornstarch and add it to the soup. Add the tomatoes and boil.

5. Simmer over low heat for ten minutes or until thickened. Add salt and pepper to taste.

Nutritional Information (per serving):

Kcal	Carbs	Protein	Fat	Sugar	Fiber
234	35g	8g	9g	9g	9g

Speedy Chicken and Meat Stews

In this sub-chapter, we explore delicious and satisfying chicken and meat stews that can be prepared in no time. These hearty dishes are packed with flavor and make for comforting meals on busy days. Whether you're craving the aromatic spices of a Moroccan tagine or the rich flavors of a classic beef stew, these recipes will help you create satisfying meals without spending hours in the kitchen.

Note: Cooking times may vary depending on the thickness of the poultry or meat, so adjust accordingly and ensure they are cooked through before serving.

Moroccan Chicken Tagine

 30'   2

Ingredients

2 tablespoons olive oil
4 chicken thighs, bone-in and skin-on
1 onion, diced
2 carrots, sliced
2 garlic cloves, minced
1 teaspoon ground cumin
1 teaspoon ground coriander
1 teaspoon ground paprika
1/2 teaspoon ground turmeric
1/4 teaspoon ground cinnamon
1 cup canned diced tomatoes
1 cup chicken broth
1/4 cup green olives, pitted
1/4 cup dried apricots, chopped
Salt and pepper to taste and fresh cilantro or parsley, chopped, for garnish

1. In a big saucepan or Dutch oven, heat the olive oil over medium-high heat.

2. Sprinkle the chicken thighs with salt and pepper before placing them skin-side down in the pot. Cook for approximately 5 minutes, or until the skin is crispy and brown. Cook the chicken thighs for a further 3 minutes after flipping. The chicken should be taken out of the pot and placed aside.

3. Place the diced onion and sliced carrots in the same saucepan. Vegetables should be sautéed for around 5 minutes until they start to soften.

4. Add the ground cinnamon, ground paprika, ground cumin, ground coriander, and ground turmeric to the saucepan. After thoroughly mixing the spices into the veggies, simmer for one more minute, or until the spices are aromatic.

5. Return the chicken thighs to the pot and add the diced tomatoes, chicken broth, green olives, and dried apricots. Stir well to combine.

6. Bring the mixture to a boil, then reduce the heat to low. Cover the pot and simmer for about 20 minutes until the chicken is cooked through and tender.

Nutritional Information (per serving):

Kcal	Carbs	Protein	Fat	Sugar	Fiber
424	14g	23g	30g	7g	2g

Spicy Beef and Vegetable Stew

 30' 2

Ingredients:

1 tablespoon olive oil	1/4 teaspoon cayenne
10 ounces beef stew	pepper (adjust to
meat, cut into bite-	taste)
sized pieces	1 can (7 ounces)
1 onion, diced	diced tomatoes
2 carrots, sliced	2 cups beef broth
2 celery stalks, sliced	1 cup frozen corn
3 garlic cloves,	kernels
minced	1 cup frozen green
1 teaspoon ground	peas
cumin	Salt and pepper to
1 teaspoon smoked	taste
paprika	Fresh parsley,
1/2 teaspoon chili	chopped, for garnish
powder	

1. Heat the olive oil in a large pot or Dutch oven over medium-high heat.

2. Add the beef stew meat to the pan and cook, stirring occasionally, for about 5 minutes, or until browned all over. Take the meat out of the saucepan, then set it aside.

3. Place the chopped onion, carrots, and celery in the same saucepan. To begin softening, sauté the veggies for around 5 minutes.

4. Add the chili powder, cayenne pepper, chili powder, cumin powder, smoked paprika, and chopped garlic to the saucepan. After thoroughly mixing the spices into the veggies, simmer for one more minute, or until the spices are aromatic.

5. Add the diced tomatoes and beef stock to the saucepan with the beef stew meat. To blend, stir.

6. Bring the mixture to a boil before turning down the heat. For around 15 minutes, simmer the saucepan with the cover on.

7. Fill the saucepan with the frozen corn kernels and green peas. Once the veggies are soft and the flavors are blended, stir well and simmer for an additional 5 minutes. To taste, add salt and pepper to the food.

Nutritional Information (per serving):

Kcal	Carbs	Protein	Fat	Sugar	Fiber
320	22g	28g	12g	7g	5g

Mediterranean Chicken&Vegetable Stew

30' 2

Ingredients:

1 tablespoon olive oil
4 boneless, skinless chicken breasts, cut into bite-sized pieces
1 onion, diced
2 bell peppers (any color), sliced
2 zucchini, sliced
3 garlic cloves, minced
1 teaspoon dried oregano
1 teaspoon dried basil
1/2 teaspoon dried thyme
1 can (7 ounces) diced tomatoes
1 cup chicken broth
1/2 cup pitted Kalamata olives, halved
Salt and pepper
Fresh parsley

1. In a big saucepan or Dutch oven, heat the olive oil over medium-high heat.

2. Include the pieces of chicken breast in the saucepan and simmer for about 5 minutes, or until browned all over. The chicken should be taken out of the pot and placed aside.

3. Place the chopped onion, bell pepper, and zucchini in the same saucepan. To begin softening, sauté the veggies for around 5 minutes.

4. Add the dried thyme, dried basil, dried oregano, and chopped garlic to the saucepan. After thoroughly mixing the herbs into the veggies, simmer for an additional minute, or until aromatic.

5. Add the diced tomatoes and chicken stock to the saucepan with the chicken. To blend, stir. The heat should be turned down once the mixture comes to a boil. For around 15 minutes, simmer the saucepan with the cover on.

6. Fill the saucepan with the Kalamata olives. Once the chicken is well cooked and the flavors are blended, stir well and simmer for an additional 5 minutes.

Nutritional Information (per serving):

Kcal	Carbs	Protein	Fat	Sugar	Fiber
290	14g	35g	8g	8g	4g

Italian Sausage and White Bean Stew

30' 2

Ingredients:

1 tablespoon olive oil
4 Italian sausages, casings removed
1 onion, diced
2 carrots, diced
2 celery stalks, diced
3 garlic cloves, minced
1 can (7 ounces) diced tomatoes
Fresh parsley
2 cups chicken broth
1 can (7 ounces each) white beans, drained and rinsed
1 teaspoon dried rosemary
1 teaspoon dried thyme
Salt and pepper to taste

1. In a big saucepan or Dutch oven, heat the olive oil over medium heat.

2. Add the Italian sausages to the pot and cook, breaking them up with a spoon, until browned and cooked through. Remove the sausages from the pot and set them aside.

3. Include the chopped celery, carrots, and onion in the same saucepan. To begin softening, sauté the veggies for around 5 minutes.

4. Stir in the minced garlic and simmer for a further minute, or until fragrant.

5. Add the diced tomatoes and chicken stock to the saucepan along with the cooked sausages.

6. Add the white beans, dried rosemary, and dried thyme to the pot. Stir well, and season with salt and pepper to taste.

7. To enable the flavors to mingle, bring the stew to a boil and cook it for about 15 minutes.

Nutritional Information (per serving):

Kcal	Carbs	Protein	Fat	Sugar	Fiber
390	29g	21g	22g	5g	8g

Flavorful Broths and Clear Soups

In this sub-chapter, we explore the world of flavorful broths and clear soups. These light and comforting dishes are known for their simplicity and delicate flavors. Whether you're seeking a nourishing chicken broth or a refreshing vegetable-based soup, these recipes will surely satisfy your cravings. Get ready to savor the rich aromas and soothing textures of these flavorful broths and clear soups.

Classic Chicken Broth

 10'   2h   2

Ingredients

1 whole chicken
2 carrots, chopped
2 celery stalks, chopped
1 onion, quartered
4 garlic cloves, smashed
1 bay leaf
6 cups water
Salt and pepper to taste
Fresh parsley, for garnish (optional)

1. In a big saucepan, combine the chicken, carrots, celery, onion, garlic cloves, and bay leaf.

2. Pour water over the chicken, ensuring it is completely saturated.

3. Over high heat, bring the saucepan to a boil. Then, turn the heat down to a simmer for about two hours, scraping any impurities that float to the top.

4. After the chicken has cooked for two hours, take it from the pot and let it cool.

5. Strain the broth through a fine-mesh sieve into another pot or large bowl, discarding the vegetables and bay leaf.

6. Season the broth with salt and pepper to taste.

7. Shred the cooked chicken meat and add it back to the broth if desired.

Nutritional Information (per serving):

Kcal	Carbs	Protein	Fat	Sugar	Fiber
554	6g	42g	33g	3g	2g

Clear Vegetable Soup

 15'   25'   2

Ingredients:

1 tablespoon olive oil
1 onion, diced
2 carrots, diced
2 celery stalks, diced
2 garlic cloves, minced
4 cups vegetable broth
1 cup green beans, trimmed and cut into bite-sized pieces
1 cup corn kernels (fresh or frozen)
1 teaspoon dried thyme
Salt and pepper to taste
Fresh parsley, chopped, for garnish (optional)
1 cup diced tomatoes

1. In a big saucepan or Dutch oven, heat the olive oil over medium heat.

2. Include the saucepan with the diced onion, carrots, celery, and garlic. To begin softening, sauté the veggies for around 5 minutes.

3. Pour in the vegetable broth and bring it to a simmer.

4. Fill the saucepan with the chopped tomatoes, green beans, corn, dried thyme, salt, and pepper. To blend, thoroughly stir. The veggies should be tender after 20 minutes of simmering the soup.

5. Taste the food and, if necessary, add more salt and pepper to the seasoning. If preferred, top the hot, clear vegetable soup with fresh parsley before serving.

Nutritional Information (per serving):

Kcal	Carbs	Protein	Fat	Sugar	Fiber
120	20g	4g	4g	7g	4g

Miso Soup with Tofu and Vegetables

 10' 15' 2

Ingredients:

4 cups vegetable broth

3 tablespoons miso paste

1 cup diced tofu

1 cup sliced mushrooms

1 cup sliced bok choy

1 green onion, thinly sliced

1 tablespoon soy sauce

1 teaspoon sesame oil

Optional toppings: seaweed, sesame seeds

1. In a pot, bring the vegetable broth to a simmer.

2. In a small bowl, whisk together the miso paste with a bit of hot water to dissolve it.

3. Add the miso paste, diced tofu, sliced mushrooms, and sliced bok choy to the simmering broth.

4. Let the soup cook for about 10 minutes, until the vegetables are tender.

5. Stir in the green onion, soy sauce, and sesame oil.

6. Serve the miso soup hot and garnish with optional toppings like seaweed and sesame seeds.

Nutritional Information (per serving):

Kcal	Carbs	Protein	Fat	Sugar	Fiber
110	8g	9g	5g	4g	2g

Lemon Chicken Orzo Soup

 10' 20' 2

Ingredients:

4 cups chicken broth

1 boneless, skinless chicken breast, cooked and shredded

1/2 cup orzo pasta

2 carrots, diced

2 celery stalks, diced

1 small onion, diced

2 garlic cloves, minced

Juice of 1 lemon

Zest of 1 lemon

Salt and pepper to taste

Fresh dill, chopped, for garnish (optional)

1. In a pot, bring the chicken broth to a boil.

2. Add the orzo pasta and cook according to the package instructions until al dente.

3. In a separate skillet, sauté the carrots, celery, onion, and minced garlic until they begin to soften.

4. Add the cooked and shredded chicken to the skillet and cook for a few minutes to heat through.

5. Transfer the vegetable and chicken mixture to the pot with the chicken broth and orzo. Stir in the lemon juice and lemon zest. Season with salt and pepper to taste.

7. Let the soup simmer for a few more minutes to allow the flavors to meld together. Serve the lemon chicken orzo soup hot, garnished with fresh dill if desired.

Nutritional Information (per serving):

Kcal	Carbs	Protein	Fat	Sugar	Fiber
160	17g	16g	3g	5g	4g

CHAPTER 7: *Effortless Snacks and Appetizers*

For entertaining or just to enjoy a tasty bite-sized treat, we look at a range of quick snacks and appetizers in Chapter 7. This chapter is jam-packed with savory and filling alternatives that are quick and simple to make, including Mediterranean dips and spreads, excellent tapas and mezze platters, easy bruschetta and crostini, swift skewers and kebabs, and flavorful oven-baked snacks.

Mediterranean Dips and Spreads

The flavorful ingredients and vivid tastes of Mediterranean cuisine are well-known. In this section, we'll look at a range of Mediterranean-inspired spreads and dips that go great with fresh veggies, pita bread, or crackers. These dips and spreads, from traditional hummus to tangy tzatziki and delicious muhammara, are guaranteed to be a favorite at any event or as a quick and delectable snack.

Classic Hummus	Tangy Tzatziki

10' 2 15' 2

Ingredients:

1 can (10 ounces) chickpeas, drained and rinsed
2 cloves garlic, minced
3 tablespoons tahini
3 tablespoons fresh lemon juice
2 tablespoons extra virgin olive oil
1/2 teaspoon ground cumin
Salt to taste
Paprika, for garnish
Fresh parsley, for garnish

Ingredients:

1 cup Greek yogurt
1/2 cucumber, grated and squeezed to remove excess moisture
2 cloves garlic, minced
1 tablespoon fresh lemon juice
1 tablespoon extra virgin olive oil
1 tablespoon chopped fresh dill
Salt and pepper to taste

1. In a food processor, combine the chickpeas, minced garlic, tahini, lemon juice, olive oil, cumin, and a pinch of salt.

2. Process the mixture until smooth and creamy, scraping down the sides of the bowl as needed.

3. Transfer the hummus to a serving dish and garnish with a sprinkle of paprika and fresh parsley. Serve with pita bread, fresh vegetables, or crackers.

1. Greek yogurt, grated cucumber, minced garlic, lemon juice, olive oil, chopped dill, and a dash of salt and pepper should all be combined in a bowl. Gently stir all the ingredients together.

2. Taste the dish and make any necessary salt and pepper adjustments.

3. To let the flavors to mingle, place in the refrigerator for at least 30 minutes. Serve as a dip for chips, with grilled veggies or pita bread.

Nutritional Information (per serving):

Kcal	Carbs	Protein	Fat	Sugar	Fiber
180	18g	6g	10g	2g	5g

Nutritional Information (per serving):

Kcal	Carbs	Protein	Fat	Sugar	Fiber
85	4g	5g	6g	3g	1g

Roasted Red Pepper and Walnut Dip

 20' 2

Ingredients:

2 large red bell peppers	1 clove garlic, minced
1/2 cup walnuts, toasted	1/2 teaspoon ground cumin
2 tablespoons extra virgin olive oil	Salt and pepper to taste
1 tablespoon lemon juice	Fresh parsley, for garnish

1. Preheat the broiler in your oven.

2. Place the red bell peppers on a baking sheet and broil for about 10 minutes, turning occasionally, until the skins are charred and blistered.

3. Remove the peppers from the oven and transfer them to a bowl. Cover the bowl with plastic wrap and let the peppers cool for about 10 minutes.

4. Once the peppers are cool enough to handle, peel off the charred skin, remove the stems and seeds, and roughly chop the flesh.

5. In a food processor, combine the roasted red peppers, toasted walnuts, olive oil, lemon juice, minced garlic, ground cumin, salt, and pepper.

6. Process the mixture until smooth and creamy, scraping down the sides of the bowl as needed.

7. Transfer the dip to a serving dish, garnish with fresh parsley, and drizzle with a little extra olive oil. Serve with pita bread, vegetable sticks, or crackers.

Nutritional Information (per serving):

Kcal	Carbs	Protein	Fat	Sugar	Fiber
180	7g	3g	17g	4g	3g

Greek Taramasalata

 15' 2

Ingredients:

4 ounces smoked cod roe (tarama)	1 clove garlic, minced
1/2 cup bread crumbs	1 small onion, finely grated
1/2 cup extra virgin olive oil	Salt and pepper to taste
2 tablespoons lemon juice	Fresh dill, for garnish

1. Place the smoked cod roe in a bowl and mash it with a fork until smooth.

2. Add the bread crumbs, olive oil, lemon juice, minced garlic, grated onion, salt, and pepper to the bowl. Mix well to combine all the ingredients until you achieve a creamy consistency.

4. Taste the dish and make any necessary seasoning adjustments, such as adding additional salt or lemon juice. Add fresh dill to the serving plate after transferring the taramasalata there.

5. Provide breadsticks, vegetable crudités, or pita bread with your meal.

Nutritional Information (per serving):

Kcal	Carbs	Protein	Fat	Sugar	Fiber
280	14g	8g	26g	1g	1g

Spicy Muhammara

 15'   2

Ingredients:

1 cup roasted red peppers, drained
1/2 cup walnuts, toasted
1/4 cup bread crumbs
1 tablespoon lemon juice
1 tablespoon pomegranate molasses

1 teaspoon ground cumin
1/2 teaspoon smoked paprika
1/2 teaspoon red pepper flakes (adjust to taste)
Salt to taste
Extra virgin olive oil, for drizzling
Chopped fresh parsley, for garnish

1. In a food processor, combine the roasted red peppers, toasted walnuts, bread crumbs, lemon juice, pomegranate molasses, ground cumin, smoked paprika, red pepper flakes, and salt.

2. Process the mixture until smooth and well combined.

3. Taste and adjust the seasonings as desired, adding more salt, lemon juice, or red pepper flakes if desired.

4. Transfer the muhammara to a serving dish and drizzle with extra virgin olive oil.

5. Garnish with chopped fresh parsley.

6. Serve with pita bread, breadsticks, or vegetable crudités.

Nutritional Information (per serving):

Kcal	Carbs	Protein	Fat	Sugar	Fiber
195	10g	4g	15g	3g	2g

Rosemary Cream

 15'   2

Ingredients:

1 cup heavy cream
2 sprigs fresh rosemary

1 clove garlic, minced
Salt and pepper to taste

1. Heat the heavy cream in a small saucepan over medium-low heat until it begins to boil. Do not let it boil.

2. Add the rosemary sprigs and minced garlic to the simmering cream.

3. Let the mixture simmer for about 3-4 minutes to infuse the flavors of the rosemary and garlic into the cream.4. Remove the saucepan from the heat and let it cool slightly.

4. Using a fine-mesh strainer, strain the cream to remove the rosemary sprigs and garlic.

5. Season the rosemary cream with salt and pepper to taste.

6. Transfer the rosemary cream to a serving bowl or container.

7. Allow the cream to cool completely, then refrigerate it for at least 1 hour to thicken before serving.

Nutritional Information (per serving):

Kcal	Carbs	Protein	Fat	Sugar	Fiber
204	2g	2g	22g	2g	1g

Tasty Tapas and Mezze Platters

Tapas and mezze platters are a delightful way to enjoy a variety of small bites and flavors. In this sub-chapter, we'll discover an assortment of tasty tapas and mezze recipes that showcase the diverse flavors of different cuisines. From stuffed grape leaves to marinated olives, stuffed mushrooms, and more, these bite-sized treats are perfect for sharing and will impress your guests with their bold and delicious flavors.

Stuffed Grape Leaves

 30' 2

Ingredients:

1 jar of grape leaves, drained and rinsed
1 cup cooked rice
1/2 cup finely chopped fresh parsley
1/4 cup finely chopped fresh mint
1/4 cup finely chopped onion
2 tablespoons lemon juice
2 tablespoons olive oil
Salt and pepper to taste

1. Combine the cooked rice, onion, parsley, mint, lemon juice, and olive oil in a bowl. Mix thoroughly.

2. Lay a single grape leaf flat on a smooth surface. Place 1 tablespoon or more of the rice mixture in the leaf's middle.

3. To wrap the leaf firmly into a tiny cylinder, tuck the bottom of the leaf over the filling, then fold the sides inward.

4. Repeat the process with the remaining grape leaves and rice mixture.

5. Place the stuffed grape leaves in a steamer basket and steam for about 15 minutes until heated through.

6. Remove them from the steamer and let them cool slightly before serving.

Nutritional Information (per serving):

Kcal	Carbs	Protein	Fat	Sugar	Fiber
160	20g	2g	7g	2g	3g

Marinated Olives with Herbs and Citrus

 10' 2

Ingredients:

2 cups mixed olives (such as Kalamata, green, and black olives)
2 tablespoons extra virgin olive oil
2 cloves garlic, minced
1 teaspoon lemon zest
1 teaspoon orange zest
1 tablespoon chopped fresh herbs (such as thyme, rosemary, or oregano)
Pinch of red pepper flakes (optional)

1. In a bowl, combine the olives, extra virgin olive oil, minced garlic, lemon zest, orange zest, fresh herbs, and red pepper flakes (if using). Toss well to coat the olives.

2. Let the olives marinate in the refrigerator for at least 1 hour to allow the flavors to meld together.

3. Before serving, let the marinated olives come to room temperature.

4. Serve the marinated olives as part of a mezze platter or as a standalone appetizer.

Nutritional Information (per serving):

Kcal	Carbs	Protein	Fat	Sugar	Fiber
150	4g	1g	14g	1g	2g

Spinach and Feta Phyllo Triangles

 25' 20' 2

Ingredients:

2 sheets phyllo
dough, thawed
2 cups fresh spinach
leaves
1/2 cup crumbled
feta cheese

1 tablespoon olive oil
Salt and pepper to
taste
Melted butter for
brushing
2 tablespoons
chopped fresh dill

1. Line a baking sheet with parchment paper and preheat the oven to 375°F (190°C).

2. Heat the olive oil in a skillet over medium heat. Add the spinach leaves and cook for two to three minutes, or until wilted. Take it off the stove and let it cool.

3. Combine the sautéed spinach, feta cheese crumbles, chopped dill, salt, and pepper in a bowl. Mix thoroughly.

4. Take one sheet of phyllo dough and brush it lightly with melted butter. Place another sheet on top and repeat the process until you have 4 layers.

5. Cut the phyllo stack into 4 equal strips.

6. Spoon about 1 tablespoon of the spinach and feta mixture onto the bottom of each strip.

7. Fold one corner of the strip over the filling to form a triangle. Continue folding the strip, maintaining the triangle shape, until you reach the end. Brush the top with melted butter to seal.

8. Carry out the procedure once more with the leftover filling and phyllo dough.

9. Place the phyllo triangles on the prepared baking sheet and bake for 15-20 minutes until golden and crispy. Remove from the oven and let them cool slightly before serving

Nutritional Information (per serving):

Kcal	Carbs	Protein	Fat	Sugar	Fiber
220	21g	6g	12g	1g	2g

Roasted Red Pepper Hummus

 10' x

Ingredients:

1 can (15 ounces) chickpeas, drained and rinsed	1 garlic clove, minced
	2 tablespoons extra virgin olive oil
1 roasted red pepper, peeled and seeded	1/2 teaspoon ground cumin
2 tablespoons tahini	Salt and pepper to taste
2 tablespoons lemon juice	Chopped fresh parsley for garnish

1. In a food processor, combine the chickpeas, roasted red pepper, tahini, lemon juice, minced garlic, olive oil, ground cumin, salt, and pepper. Blend until smooth and creamy.

2. Taste and adjust the seasonings as needed.

3. Transfer the roasted red pepper hummus to a serving bowl.

4. Drizzle with a little extra virgin olive oil and sprinkle with chopped fresh parsley for garnish.

5. Serve the roasted red pepper hummus with pita bread, fresh vegetables, or as a dip for your favorite snacks.

Nutritional Information (per serving):

Kcal	Carbs	Protein	Fat	Sugar	Fiber
160	16g	6g	11g	2g	5g

Grilled Halloumi Skewers with Lemon and Herbs

 15' 10' 2

Ingredients:

8 ounces halloumi cheese, cut into cubes	1 tablespoon chopped fresh herbs (such as oregano, thyme, or rosemary)
1 lemon, zested and juiced	
2 tablespoons extra virgin olive oil	Salt and pepper to taste
	Wooden skewers, soaked in water for 30 minutes

1. Preheat a grill or grill pan over medium-high heat.

2. In a bowl, combine the lemon zest, lemon juice, olive oil, chopped herbs, salt, and pepper. Mix well.

3. Thread the halloumi cheese cubes onto the soaked wooden skewers.

4. Brush the halloumi skewers with the lemon and herb mixture, making sure to coat all sides.

5. Place the halloumi skewers on the preheated grill and cook for about 3-4 minutes on each side, until grill marks appear and the cheese is softened and slightly charred.

6. Remove the skewers from the grill and let them cool slightly before serving.

7. Serve the grilled halloumi skewers with lemon and herbs as a tasty appetizer or part of a mezze platter.

Nutritional Information (per serving):

Kcal	Carbs	Protein	Fat	Sugar	Fiber
240	3g	13g	23g	3g	1g

Easy Bruschetta and Crostini

It is possible to add different toppings to the traditional appetizers, bruschetta and crostini, to suit your preferences. We'll look at simple bruschetta and crostini recipes that are flavorful and easy to make in this subsection. These snacks range from the classic tomato and basil bruschetta to inventive pairings like fig and goat cheese crostini, roasted red pepper and feta crostini, and more. They are suitable for any occasion.

Tomato and Basil Bruschetta	Fig and Goat Cheese Crostini

 10 min   2

 15'   2

Ingredients:

4 slices of crusty bread	2 tablespoons extra-virgin olive oil
2 ripe tomatoes, diced	1 garlic clove, minced
1/4 cup fresh basil leaves, chopped	Salt and pepper to taste

1. Preheat your oven to 350°F (175°C).

2. Place the bread slices on a baking sheet and toast them in the oven until lightly golden and crispy.

3. In a bowl, combine the diced tomatoes, chopped basil, minced garlic, olive oil, salt, and pepper. Mix well.

4. Remove the toasted bread from the oven and let it cool slightly.

5. Spoon the tomato and basil mixture onto each bread slice, spreading it evenly.

Nutritional Information (per serving):

Kcal	Carbs	Protein	Fat	Sugar	Fiber
120	16g	4g	6g	3g	2g

Ingredients:

4 slices of baguette	2 tablespoons honey
4 fresh figs, sliced	Fresh thyme leaves
4 ounces goat cheese	for garnish

1. Preheat your oven to 350°F (175°C).

2. Place the baguette slices on a baking sheet and toast them in the oven until lightly crisp.

3. Spread a generous layer of goat cheese on each toasted slice.

4. Top each slice with sliced figs, drizzle with honey, and sprinkle with fresh thyme leaves.

Nutritional Information (per serving):

Kcal	Carbs	Protein	Fat	Sugar	Fiber
160	25g	6g	6g	14g	3g

Roasted Red Pepper and Feta Crostini

 20' 2

Ingredients:

4 slices of rustic bread
1 roasted red pepper, sliced
2 ounces feta cheese, crumbled

1 tablespoon balsamic glaze
Fresh basil leaves for garnish

1. Preheat your oven to 350°F (175°C).

2. Place the bread slices on a baking sheet and toast them in the oven until lightly golden.

3. Arrange the roasted red pepper slices on top of each toasted slice. Sprinkle crumbled feta cheese over the peppers. Drizzle balsamic glaze over the crostini. Garnish with fresh basil leaves.

Nutritional Information (per serving):

Kcal	Carbs	Protein	Fat	Sugar	Fiber
180	22g	7g	7g	5g	2g

Artichoke and Parmesan Bruschetta

 20' 2

Ingredients:

4 slices of Italian bread
1 can (7 ounces) artichoke hearts, drained and chopped
1/2 cup grated Parmesan cheese

2 tablespoons mayonnaise
1 tablespoon lemon juice
1 garlic clove, minced
Fresh parsley for garnish

1. Preheat your oven to 350°F (175°C).

2. Place the bread slices on a baking sheet and toast them in the oven until they are crispy, about 8-10 minutes.

3. In a bowl, mix together the chopped artichoke hearts, grated Parmesan cheese, mayonnaise, lemon juice, and minced garlic.

4. Remove the toasted bread from the oven and let it cool slightly.

5. Spread the artichoke mixture onto each bread slice, spreading it evenly.

6. Place the bruschetta back in the oven for an additional 5 minutes until the topping is heated through and slightly melted.

7. Garnish with fresh parsley.

8. Serve immediately and enjoy!

Nutritional Information (per serving):

Kcal	Carbs	Protein	Fat	Sugar	Fiber
180	20g	9g	8g	1g	5g

Caramelized Onion and Brie Crostini

 20' 2

Ingredients:

4 slices of baguette
2 large onions, thinly sliced
2 tablespoons butter
1 tablespoon brown sugar

4 ounces Brie cheese, sliced
Fresh thyme leaves for garnish
Salt and pepper to taste

1. Set the oven temperature to 375°F (190°C).

2. Arrange the bread pieces on a baking sheet and toast them in the oven until they are crisp and just beginning to turn golden, about 5-7 minutes.

3. Melt the butter in a large pan over medium heat. After adding the onions, simmer them for approximately 15 minutes, turning regularly, until they are caramelized and golden brown.

4. Sprinkle brown sugar over the caramelized onions and stir until it is dissolved. Spread a layer of caramelized onions onto each toasted bread slice.

6. Top with sliced Brie cheese and sprinkle fresh thyme leaves on top.

7. Place the topped crostini back in the oven for another 5 minutes to melt the cheese. Serve the caramelized onion and Brie crostini as a rich and savory appetizer.

Nutritional Information (per serving):

Kcal	Carbs	Protein	Fat	Sugar	Fiber
280	28g	9g	13g	8g	2g

Caprese Bruschetta

 15' 2

Ingredients:

4 slices of Italian bread
2 ripe tomatoes, sliced
4 ounces fresh mozzarella cheese, sliced

Fresh basil leaves
2 tablespoons balsamic glaze
Salt and pepper to taste

1. Preheat the oven to 375°F (190°C).

2. Place the bread slices on a baking sheet and toast in the oven for about 5-7 minutes until they are crispy and lightly golden.

3. Arrange tomato slices on each toasted bread slice.

4. Top with slices of fresh mozzarella cheese

5. Place a few fresh basil leaves on top of the cheese.

6. Drizzle balsamic glaze over the bruschetta.

7. Season with salt and pepper to taste.

8. Serve the Caprese bruschetta as a refreshing and flavorful appetizer.

Nutritional Information (per serving):

Kcal	Carbs	Protein	Fat	Sugar	Fiber
230	25g	12g	8g	8g	3g

Speedy Skewers and Kebabs

A tasty and entertaining method to consume bite-sized pieces of meat, fish, or veggies is with skewers and kebabs. In this chapter, we'll learn about simple skewer and kebab dishes that are ideal for quick and filling snacks or party appetizers. These recipes range from marinated chicken skewers to grilled shrimp kebabs and veggie skewers, and they may be baked, grilled, or stovetop cooked.

Teriyaki Chicken Skewers

 20' 10' 30' 2

Ingredients:

1 pound boneless, skinless chicken breasts, cut into bite-sized pieces	1 teaspoon grated fresh ginger
1/4 cup soy sauce	1 bell pepper, cut into chunks
2 tablespoons honey	1 red onion, cut into chunks
1 tablespoon rice vinegar	Salt and pepper to taste
1 tablespoon sesame oil	Sesame seeds for garnish (optional)
1 clove garlic, minced	Green onions, chopped, for garnish (optional)

1. To create the teriyaki marinade, combine the soy sauce, honey, rice vinegar, sesame oil, chopped garlic, and grated ginger in a basin.

2. Spread the teriyaki marinade over the chicken pieces and place them in a shallow dish. Toss to evenly coat the chicken. Refrigerate the marinade for at least 30 minutes.

3. Heat the grill or grill pan to a high temperature. Alternating the ingredients, thread the marinated chicken, bell pepper pieces, and red onion chunks onto skewers, grill the skewers for 8 to 10 minutes, flipping once.

4. Add salt and pepper to the skewers. Until the chicken is well cooked and faintly

5. Remove the skewers from the grill and garnish with sesame seeds and chopped green onions, if desired.

6. Serve the teriyaki chicken skewers as a delicious and satisfying appetizer.

Nutritional Information (per serving):

Kcal	Carbs	Protein	Fat	Sugar	Fiber
230	15g	27g	7g	12g	2g

Shrimp and Pineapple Skewers

 15' 10' 30' 2

Ingredients:

12 ounces large shrimp, peeled and deveined
1 cup pineapple chunks
2 tablespoons olive oil
2 tablespoons soy sauce

2 tablespoons honey
1 tablespoon lime juice
1 teaspoon chili powder
Salt and pepper to taste
Fresh cilantro leaves for garnish (optional)

1. In a bowl, whisk together olive oil, soy sauce, honey, lime juice, chili powder, salt, and pepper to make the marinade.

2. Place the shrimp and pineapple chunks in a shallow dish, and pour the marinade over them. Toss to coat evenly. Marinate for 30 minutes in the refrigerator.

3. Preheat the grill or grill pan over medium-high heat.

4. Thread the marinated shrimp and pineapple onto skewers, alternating the ingredients.

5. Season the skewers with salt and pepper.

6. Grill the skewers for about 2-3 minutes per side until the shrimp are pink and cooked through.

7. Remove the skewers from the grill and garnish with fresh cilantro leaves, if desired.

Nutritional Information (per serving):

Kcal	Carbs	Protein	Fat	Sugar	Fiber
190	16g	21g	6g	13g	1g

Beef and Vegetable Kebabs

 20' 10' 30' 2

Ingredients:

12 ounces beef sirloin, cut into 1-inch cubes
1 bell pepper, cut into chunks
1 red onion, cut into chunks
8-10 cherry tomatoes
2 tablespoons olive oil

2 tablespoons balsamic vinegar
2 cloves garlic, minced
1 teaspoon dried oregano
Salt and pepper to taste
Fresh parsley leaves for garnish (optional)

1. In a bowl, whisk together olive oil, balsamic vinegar, minced garlic, dried oregano, salt, and pepper to make the marinade.

2. Place the beef cubes, bell pepper chunks, red onion chunks, and cherry tomatoes in a shallow dish and pour the marinade over them. Toss to coat evenly. Marinate for 30 minutes in the refrigerator.

3. Preheat the grill or grill pan over medium-high heat. Thread the marinated beef, bell pepper, red onion, and cherry tomatoes onto skewers, alternating the ingredients.

4. Season the skewers with salt and pepper. Grill the skewers for about 10-12 minutes, turning occasionally, until the beef is cooked to your desired level of doneness.

5. Remove the skewers from the grill and garnish with fresh parsley leaves, if desired.

Nutritional Information (per serving):

Kcal	Carbs	Protein	Fat	Sugar	Fiber
260	11g	26g	13g	6g	2g

Flavorful Oven-Baked Snacks

Treats cooked in the oven still have a ton of taste and crunch while being a healthier alternative to deep-fried treats. We'll look at a variety of delectable oven-baked snacks in this section that are ideal for sating your snacking desires. These snacks range from cheese-filled baked spinach balls to smoky roasted chickpeas, are easy to make, and can be eaten guilt-free.

Parmesan Baked Zucchini Fries	Spicy Baked Chickpeas

 15' 20' 2   10' 30' 2

Ingredients:

2 medium zucchini, cut into fries-like strips
1 cup breadcrumbs
1 teaspoon dried oregano

½ teaspoon garlic powder
2 eggs, lightly beaten
Salt and pepper to taste
½ cup grated Parmesan cheese

1. Set the oven temperature to 425°F (220°C). Cooking spray should be sparingly used after lining a baking sheet with parchment paper.

2. Combine the breadcrumbs, Parmesan cheese, dried oregano, garlic powder, salt, and pepper in a shallow plate.

3. Coat each zucchini strip in the breadcrumb mixture after dipping it into the beaten eggs, letting any excess drop off. The breadcrumbs need to be softly pressed to stick.

4. Arrange the coated zucchini strips in a single layer on the baking sheet that has been prepared. Bake for 15 to 20 minutes, or until the zucchini fries are crisp and golden brown, in the preheated oven.

5. Take them out of the oven and give them a little cooling period before serving.

Nutritional Information (per serving):

Kcal	Carbs	Protein	Fat	Sugar	Fiber
160	17g	10g	6g	3g	3g

Ingredients:

1 can (10 ounces) chickpeas, drained and rinsed
2 tablespoons olive oil
1 teaspoon smoked paprika
1/2 teaspoon cayenne pepper

1/2 teaspoon garlic powder
1/2 teaspoon salt
Fresh cilantro or parsley for garnish (optional)

1. Preheat the oven to 400°F (200°C). Line a baking sheet with parchment paper.

2. In a bowl, toss the chickpeas with olive oil, smoked paprika, cayenne pepper, garlic powder, and salt until they are evenly coated.

3. Spread the seasoned chickpeas in a single layer on the prepared baking sheet.

4. Bake in the preheated oven for 25-30 minutes, stirring once or twice during baking, until the chickpeas are crispy and golden brown.

5. Remove them from the oven and let them cool for a few minutes.

6. Serve the spicy baked chickpeas as a flavorful and protein-packed snack.

Nutritional Information (per serving):

Kcal	Carbs	Protein	Fat	Sugar	Fiber
190	24g	8g	7g	4g	7g

Baked Pita Chips

 10' 15' 2

Ingredients:

4 pita bread rounds
2 tablespoons olive oil
1 teaspoon dried oregano

½ teaspoon garlic powder
Salt and pepper to taste

1. Set the oven temperature to 375°F (190°C). Use parchment paper to cover a baking sheet.

2. Cut each pita bread round into 8 wedges.

3. In a small bowl, mix together the olive oil, dried oregano, garlic powder, salt, and pepper.

4. Brush both sides of each pita wedge with the olive oil mixture and place them in a single layer on the prepared baking sheet.

5. Bake in the preheated oven for 12-15 minutes, or until the pita chips are golden brown and crispy. Remove them from the oven and let them cool before serving.

7. Serve the baked pita chips with your favorite dips or enjoy them on their own as a crunchy and flavorful snack.

Nutritional Information (per serving):

Kcal	Carbs	Protein	Fat	Sugar	Fiber
150	20g	4g	5g	1g	2g

Crispy Baked Kale Chips

 10' 15' 2

Ingredients:

1 bunch kale
1 tablespoon olive oil
1/2 teaspoon salt

1/2 teaspoon garlic powder
1/4 teaspoon paprika

1. Preheat the oven to 350°F (175°C). Line a baking sheet with parchment paper.

2. Wash and dry the kale thoroughly. Remove the tough stems and tear the leaves into bite-sized pieces.

3. In a large bowl, toss the kale with olive oil, salt, garlic powder, and paprika. Ensure that the leaves are evenly coated with the seasoning.

4. On the prepared baking sheet, arrange the seasoned kale leaves in a single layer.

5. Bake the kale chips in the preheated oven for 12 to 15 minutes, or until crisp and lightly browned. Watch them closely to avoid scorching them.

6. Take them out of the oven and allow them to cool before serving.

7. Snack on the crunchy baked kale chips for a guilt-free and healthful choice.

Nutritional Information (per serving):

Kcal	Carbs	Protein	Fat	Sugar	Fiber
70	7g	3g	4g	2g	3g

CHAPTER 8: *Quick and Healthy Desserts*

With these simple and nutritious dessert recipes, you can indulge in delicious and guilt-free sweets. There is something for everyone to satiate their sweet craving, from scrumptious baked fruit crisps to cool fruit salads. These dishes are created to be simple, nourishing, and flavorful, whether you're searching for a tasty energy bite or a light and fruity dessert.

Speedy Baked Fruit Crisps

Apple Cinnamon Crisp	Peach and Blueberry Crisp

 10' 30' 2   15' 35' 2

Apple Cinnamon Crisp

Ingredients:

4 cups sliced apples
2 tablespoons lemon juice
1/4 cup maple syrup
1 teaspoon ground cinnamon
1/2 cup rolled oats

1/4 cup almond flour
1/4 cup chopped nuts (e.g., walnuts, pecans)
2 tablespoons coconut oil, melted

1. Preheat the oven to 350°F (175°C).

2. In a large bowl, toss the sliced apples with lemon juice, maple syrup, and ground cinnamon.

3. In a separate bowl, combine rolled oats, almond flour, chopped nuts, and melted coconut oil. Stir until well mixed and crumbly.

4. Spread the apple mixture evenly in a baking dish. Sprinkle the oat-nut mixture over the apples, covering them completely.

5. Bake in the preheated oven for 30 minutes, or until the apples are tender and the topping is golden brown.

6. Remove it from the oven and let it cool slightly before serving.

Nutritional Information (per serving):

Kcal	Carbs	Protein	Fat	Sugar	Fiber
290	38g	4g	15g	23g	5g

Peach and Blueberry Crisp

Ingredients:

4 cups sliced peaches
1 cup blueberries
2 tablespoons lemon juice
1/4 cup honey or maple syrup
1 teaspoon vanilla extract

1/2 cup rolled oats
1/4 cup almond flour
1/4 cup chopped almonds
2 tablespoons coconut oil, melted

1. Preheat the oven to 350°F (175°C).

2. In a large bowl, combine sliced peaches, blueberries, lemon juice, honey or maple syrup, and vanilla extract. Mix well to coat the fruit.

3. In a separate bowl, mix rolled oats, almond flour, chopped almonds, and melted coconut oil until crumbly.

4. Transfer the fruit mixture to a baking dish. Sprinkle the oat-almond mixture evenly over the fruit.

5. Bake in the preheated oven for 35 minutes, or until the fruit is bubbling and the topping is golden brown. Remove it from the oven and let it cool slightly before serving.

Nutritional Information (per serving):

Kcal	Carbs	Protein	Fat	Sugar	Fiber
270	46g	6g	9g	33g	6g

Mixed Berry Oatmeal Crisp

 15' 30' 2

Ingredients:

2 cups mixed berries (e.g., strawberries, raspberries, blackberries)
2 tablespoons lemon juice
¼ cup honey or maple syrup
1 teaspoon vanilla extract

1 cup rolled oats
¼ cup almond flour
¼ cup chopped pecans or walnuts
2 tablespoons coconut oil, melted
Optional: Greek yogurt or vanilla ice cream for serving

1. Preheat the oven to 350°F (175°C).

2. In a bowl, toss the mixed berries with lemon juice, honey or maple syrup, and vanilla extract.

3. In a separate bowl, combine rolled oats, almond flour, chopped pecans or walnuts, and melted coconut oil. Mix until crumbly.

4. Place the mixed berries in a baking dish. Sprinkle the oat-nut mixture over the berries, covering them evenly.

5. Bake in the preheated oven for 30 minutes, or until the fruit is bubbly and the topping is golden brown.

6. Remove it from the oven and let it cool slightly before serving.

7. Serve warm with a dollop of Greek yogurt or a scoop of vanilla ice cream, if desired.

Nutritional Information (per serving):

Kcal	Carbs	Protein	Fat	Sugar	Fiber
260	43g	5g	9g	22g	5g

Mango Coconut Crisp

 15' 30' 2

Ingredients:

4 cups sliced mangoes
2 tablespoons lime juice
1/4 cup honey or maple syrup
1/2 cup shredded coconut

1/4 cup almond flour
1/4 cup chopped macadamia nuts
2 tablespoons coconut oil, melted
Optional: Coconut whipped cream or vanilla ice cream for serving

1. Preheat the oven to 350°F (175°C).

2. In a large bowl, combine the sliced mangoes, lime juice, and honey or maple syrup. Mix well to coat the mangoes.

3. In a separate bowl, mix shredded coconut, almond flour, chopped macadamia nuts, and melted coconut oil until crumbly.

4. Transfer the mango mixture to a baking dish. Sprinkle the coconut-nut mixture evenly over the mangoes.

5. Bake in the preheated oven for 30 minutes, or until the mangoes are tender and the topping is golden brown.

6. Remove it from the oven and let it cool slightly before serving.

7. If preferred, top the warm dish with a scoop of vanilla ice cream or a dollop of coconut whipped cream.

Nutritional Information (per serving):

Kcal	Carbs	Protein	Fat	Sugar	Fiber
410	46g	4g	26g	41g	5g

Pear and Cranberry Crisp

 15' 35' 2

Ingredients:

4 cups sliced pears
1 cup fresh or frozen cranberries
2 tablespoons lemon juice
1/4 cup honey or maple syrup
1 teaspoon ground cinnamon

1/2 cup rolled oats
1/4 cup almond flour
1/4 cup chopped walnuts
2 tablespoons coconut oil, melted
Optional: Vanilla yogurt or whipped cream for serving

1. Preheat the oven to 350°F (175°C).

2. In a large bowl, combine the sliced pears, cranberries, lemon juice, honey or maple syrup, and ground cinnamon. Mix well to coat the fruit.

3. In a separate bowl, mix rolled oats, almond flour, chopped walnuts, and melted coconut oil until crumbly.

4. Transfer the fruit mixture to a baking dish. Sprinkle the oat-nut mixture evenly over the fruit.

5. Bake in the preheated oven for 35 minutes, or until the fruit is tender and the topping is golden brown.

6. Remove it from the oven and let it cool slightly before serving.

7. Serve warm with a dollop of vanilla yogurt or whipped cream, if desired.

Nutritional Information (per serving):

Kcal	Carbs	Protein	Fat	Sugar	Fiber
270	49g	4g	11g	36g	7g

Mediterranean-Inspired Sweet Pastries

Orange Blossom Scented Semolina Cake

 20' 35' 4

Ingredients:

1 cup fine semolina
1 cup plain yogurt
1 cup granulated sugar
1 cup unsalted butter, melted
1 cup all-purpose flour
1 teaspoon baking powder

1/4 cup orange blossom water
Zest of 1 orange
Syrup:
1 cup granulated sugar
1 cup water
Juice of 1 lemon
1 teaspoon vanilla extract

1. Preheat the oven to 350°F (175°C).

2. In a mixing bowl, combine the semolina, yogurt, granulated sugar, melted butter, flour, baking powder, vanilla extract, orange blossom water, and orange zest. Mix well until all the ingredients are incorporated.

3. Grease a baking dish with butter or cooking spray. Pour the batter into the dish and spread it evenly.

4. Bake in the preheated oven for about 35 minutes, or until the cake is golden brown and a toothpick inserted into the center comes out clean.

5. Make the syrup while the cake is baking. Lemon juice, water, and granulated sugar should all be combined in a pot. The mixture should be heated until it boils, then it should be simmered for ten minutes.

6. Once the cake is out of the oven, immediately pour the hot syrup over it, ensuring that it covers the entire cake. Serve at room temperature

Nutritional Information (per serving):

Kcal	Carbs	Protein	Fat	Sugar	Fiber
1387	113g	10g	47g	57g	2g

Italian Cannoli

 30'   10'   4

Ingredients:

1 cup all-purpose flour	Pinch of salt
2 tablespoons granulated sugar	Vegetable oil for frying
2 tablespoons unsalted butter, melted	1 cup ricotta cheese
1/4 cup Marsala wine	1/2 cup powdered sugar
1/4 teaspoon ground cinnamon	1/4 cup chopped pistachios
	Chocolate chips or grated chocolate, for garnish

1. In a mixing bowl, combine the flour, granulated sugar, melted butter, Marsala wine, ground cinnamon, and salt. Mix until a dough forms.

2. Knead the dough on a lightly floured surface until it becomes smooth and elastic.

3. Cover the dough with plastic wrap and let it rest in the refrigerator for about 1 hour.

4. Heat vegetable oil in a deep saucepan or fryer to approximately 350°F (175°C).

5. Roll out the dough thinly on a floured surface and cut it into circles using a round cookie cutter or a glass.

6. Wrap each dough circle around a cannoli tube or a metal cannoli form, sealing the edges with a little water.

7. Fry the cannoli shells in the hot oil until golden brown and crispy. Remove them from the oil and let them cool on a wire rack.

8. In a bowl, mix the ricotta cheese and powdered sugar until smooth and creamy.

9. Fill a piping bag with the ricotta mixture and pipe it into both ends of each cooled cannoli shell.

10. Dip the ends of the filled cannoli in the chopped pistachios and sprinkle with chocolate chips or grated chocolate.

11. Refrigerate the cannoli for at least 50/60 minutes before serving to allow the filling to set.

12. Serve the Italian cannoli chilled, and enjoy!

Nutritional Information (per serving):

Kcal	Carbs	Protein	Fat	Sugar	Fiber
430	55g	9g	18g	24g	2g

Nutritious Energy Balls and Bites

We delve into the realm of wholesome energy balls and nibbles in the next section. These tasty bite-sized snacks offer a rapid boost of nutrition and energy and are made with all-natural ingredients. These dishes will sate your desires and keep you fueled, whether you need a mid-day pick-me-up or a post-workout boost. Prepare to savor a range of tastes and textures that will have you wanting more!

Almond Coconut Energy Balls

 15'   10 balls

Ingredients:

1 cup almond flour
1/2 cup shredded coconut
1/4 cup almond butter
2 tablespoons honey or maple syrup

1/2 teaspoon vanilla extract
Pinch of salt
Optional: extra shredded coconut for rolling

1. In a mixing bowl, combine the almond flour, shredded coconut, almond butter, honey or maple syrup, vanilla extract, and salt. Mix well until the ingredients are fully incorporated.

2. Roll the mixture into small balls, about 1 inch in diameter.

3. Optional: Roll the energy balls in shredded coconut for an extra coating.

4. Place the energy balls in an airtight container and refrigerate for at least 1 hour to firm up.

5. Serve chilled and enjoy these delightful almond and coconut energy balls!

Nutritional Information (per energy ball):

Kcal	Carbs	Protein	Fat	Sugar	Fiber
386	21g	9g	32g	11g	7g

Peanut Butter Chocolate Chip Bites

 20'   10 bites

Ingredients:

1 cup rolled oats
1/2 cup natural peanut butter
1/4 cup honey or maple syrup
Pinch of salt

1/4 cup mini chocolate chips
1/4 cup chopped nuts (e.g., almonds, walnuts)
1/4 teaspoon vanilla extract

1. In a food processor, pulse the rolled oats until they become a coarse flour-like consistency.

2. In a mixing bowl, combine the oat flour, peanut butter, honey or maple syrup, mini chocolate chips, chopped nuts, vanilla extract, and salt. Mix well until all the ingredients are evenly distributed.

3. Form bite-sized balls out of the mixture using tiny amounts.

4. Arrange the chocolate chip bits with peanut butter on a baking sheet covered with parchment paper.

5. To firm up, place the bites in the fridge for at least 30 minutes.

Nutritional Information (per bite):

Kcal	Carbs	Protein	Fat	Sugar	Fiber
446	50g	13g	25g	24g	7g

Coconut Lime Energy Bites

 20'   10 bites

Ingredients:

1 cup unsweetened shredded coconut	2 tablespoons lime juice
1/2 cup raw cashews	2 tablespoons honey or maple syrup
1/4 cup dates, pitted	1/2 teaspoon vanilla extract
Zest of 1 lime	
Pinch of sal	

1. In a food processor, blend the shredded coconut, raw cashews, pitted dates, lime zest, lime juice, honey or maple syrup, vanilla extract, and salt until a sticky mixture forms.

2. Form bite-sized balls out of the mixture using tiny amounts.

3. Place the coconut-lime energy bites on a plate or baking sheet.

4. Refrigerate the bites for at least 1 hour to firm up.

5. Serve chilled and enjoy the tropical flavors of these coconut lime energy bites!

Nutritional Information (per bite):

Kcal	Carbs	Protein	Fat	Sugar	Fiber
360	31g	5g	27g	17g	6g

Chocolate Almond Protein Balls

 15'   10 balls

Ingredients:

1 cup almond meal	2 tablespoons honey or maple syrup
1/4 cup unsweetened cocoa powder	1 teaspoon vanilla extract
1/4 cup chocolate protein powder	Pinch of salt
1/4 cup almond butter	

1. In a mixing bowl, combine the almond meal, cocoa powder, chocolate protein powder, almond butter, honey or maple syrup, vanilla extract, and salt. Mix well until the ingredients are fully incorporated.

2. Take small portions of the mixture and roll them into balls.

3. Place the chocolate almond protein balls on a plate or baking sheet.

4. Refrigerate the balls for at least 30 minutes to firm them up.

5. Serve chilled and enjoy these protein-packed chocolate treats!

Nutritional Information (per ball):

Kcal	Carbs	Protein	Fat	Sugar	Fiber
306	20g	13g	21g	11g	6g

CHAPTER 9: *Meal Plans Menus*

DAYS	BREAKFAST	LUNCH	DINNER
1	Mediterranean Eggs and Ricotta Cheese	Mediterranean Carrot Onion and Ricotta Cheese Soup	Avocado and Tuna Tapas
2	Fruit Yogurt	Turkey Breast with Fava Bean and Artichoke Heart Salad	Roasted Chicken Breast Fillet with Kalamata Olives and Capers
3	Savory Breakfast Oatmeal	Bulgur Pilaf with Roasted Red Bell Peppers	Simple and Easy Turkey Breast Fillet Wraps
4	Avocado Tomato and Egg	Mediterranean Chickpea and Grape Salad	Mango and Coconut Frozen Pie
5	Baked Eggs with Cottage Cheese	Tomato Basil Pasta	Baked Lamb Chops
6	Crustless Tiropita	Ritzy Veggie Chili	Pecan and Carrot Cake
7	Mediterranean Vegetable Omelet	Caprese Fusilli	Zucchini and Artichokes Bowl with Farro
8	Berry and Nut Parfait	Walnut and Ricotta Spaghetti	Garlicky Zucchini Cubes with Mint
9	Kale and Apple Smoothie	Chard and Mushroom Risotto	Parsley-Dijon Chicken and Potatoes
10	Calo Cinnamon Oatmeal	Pesto Pasta	Cauliflower Hash with Carrots
11	Fruit Yogurt	One-Pot Mushroom Risotto	Lemon Garlic Shrimp Skewers
12	Avocado Toast with Goat Cheese	Garlic Shrimp Fettuccine	Sweet Potato and Tomato Curry
13	Banana-Blueberry Breakfast Cookies	Lentil Risotto	Macadamia Pork
14	Blackberry-Yogurt Green Smoothie	Cheesy Tomato Linguine	Glazed Mushroom and Vegetable Fajitas

15	Spinach Cheese Pie	Spaghetti Ragù Bolognese	Spicy Tofu Tacos with Cherry Tomato Salsa
16	Baked Ricotta with Honey Pears	Black Bean Chili with Mangoes	Roasted Tomato Panini
17	Pancakes with Berry Sauce	Italian Sautéed Cannellini Beans	Vegetable and Cheese Lavash Pizza
18	Apple-Tahini Toast	Cumin Quinoa Pilaf	Lamb Tagine with Couscous and Almonds
19	Tomato and Egg Breakfast Pizza	Grana Padano Risotto	Cheesy Sweet Potato Burgers
20	Avocado and Egg Toast	Mint Brown Rice	Cauliflower Rice Risotto with Mushrooms
21	Tropical Paradise Smoothie Bowl	Mediterranean Lemon Garlic Pasta	Baked Salmon with Basil and Tomato
22	Creamy Vanilla Oatmeal	Farro Salad with Roasted Vegetables	Spiced Roast Chicken
23	Mediterranean Citrus Smoothie	Bulgur Salad with Chickpeas and Herbs	Lemony Shrimp with Orzo Salad
24	Healthy Chia Pudding	Lentil and Vegetable Curry Stew	Grilled Chicken and Zucchini Kebabs
25	Feta and Spinach Frittata	Wild Rice, Celery, and Cauliflower Pilaf	Roasted Chicken Thighs With Basmati
26	Protein-Packed Almond Butter Smoothie	Seashell Pasta with Shrimp and Cherry Tomatoes	Zucchini Fritters
27	Mediterranean Shakshuka	Greek Salad with Lemon-Herb Dressing	Pan-Seared Pompano Fish and Black Olive
28	Egg Bake	Roasted Ratatouille Pasta	Grilled Vegetable Skewers
29	Pumpkin Pie Parfait	Bean and Veggie Pasta	Sautéed Green Beans with Tomatoes
30	Berry Blast Smoothie	Brussels Sprouts Linguine	Chicken Breast Hummus and Feta Cheese

DAY 1

Breakfast: Mediterranean Eggs and Ricotta Cheese

 15' 2

Ingredients

4 eggs
1 cup ricotta cheese
1 cup cherry tomatoes, halved

1/4 cup chopped fresh basil
Salt and pepper to taste

1. Heat olive oil in a non-stick pan over medium heat.

2. Add diced tomatoes, chopped spinach, and minced garlic. Sauté for 2-3 minutes.

3. Add salt and pepper to the eggs as they are cracked into the pan. Cook until the eggs reach the desired doneness. Serve the eggs with a dollop of ricotta cheese on top

Nutritional information per serving:

Kcal	Carbs	Protein	Fat	Sugar	Fiber
250	5g	22g	18g	2g	1g

Lunch: Mediterranean Carrot Onion and Ricotta Cheese Soup

 25' 2

Ingredients

1 tablespoon olive oil
1 onion, chopped

4 carrots, peeled and chopped
4 cups vegetable broth

1. Heat olive oil in a large pot over medium heat.

2. Add diced onions, chopped carrots, and minced garlic. Sauté for 5 minutes until softened

.3. Add vegetable broth, dried oregano, dried thyme, and salt. Bring to a boil, then reduce heat and simmer for 20 minutes.

4. Puree the soup using an immersion blender, or transfer it to a blender and blend until smooth.

Nutritional information per serving:

Kcal	Carbs	Protein	Fat	Sugar	Fiber
190	18g	8g	9g	9g	4g

Dinner: Avocado and Tuna Tapas

 10' 2

Ingredients

2 ripe avocados, halved and pitted
1 can tuna, drained
1 tablespoon lemon juice
2 tablespoons chopped fresh parsley

Salt and pepper to taste
1 cup ricotta cheese
Salt and pepper to taste

1. In a bowl, combine canned tuna, mashed avocado, diced red onion, chopped cilantro, and freshly squeezed lemon juice.

2. Season with salt, pepper, and a pinch of cayenne pepper for a kick.

3. Mix well until all ingredients are evenly combined.

4. Slice a baguette into thin rounds and lightly toast them.

5. Spoon the avocado and tuna mixture onto each toasted baguette slice.

Nutritional information per serving:

Kcal	Carbs	Protein	Fat	Sugar	Fiber
120	5g	7g	9g	1g	5g

DAY 2

Breakfast: Fruit Yogurt

 10'   2

Ingredients

2 cups plain Greek yogurt	2 tablespoons honey
2 cups mixed fresh fruits (such as berries, sliced peaches, or diced mango)	1/4 cup chopped nuts (such as almonds or walnuts

1. In a bowl, combine your choice of Greek yogurt with a variety of fresh fruits, such as berries, sliced bananas, and diced mango.

2. Drizzle with honey or sprinkle with granola for added sweetness and crunch.

Nutritional information per serving:

Kcal	Carbs	Protein	Fat	Sugar	Fiber
250	27g	20g	9g	20g	5g

Lunch: Turkey with Fava Bean and Artichoke Salad

 20'   2

Ingredients

4 turkey breast fillets	2 tablespoons chopped fresh parsley
1 cup cooked fava beans	
1 cup artichoke hearts, quartered	2 tablespoons lemon juice
1 cup cherry tomatoes, halved	2 tablespoons olive oil
	Salt and pepper to taste

1. Season turkey breast with salt, pepper, and dried herbs of your choice.

2. Grill or pan-sear the turkey until cooked through and nicely browned on the outside.

3. In a bowl, combine cooked fava beans, marinated artichoke hearts, cherry tomatoes, and chopped fresh herbs like parsley and mint. Drizzle with olive oil and lemon juice for dressing, and toss gently to combine.

Nutritional information per serving:

Kcal	Carbs	Protein	Fat	Sugar	Fiber
320	14g	40g	12g	2g	5g

Dinner: Roasted Chicken with Olives and Capers

 25'   2

Ingredients

4 chicken breast fillets	2 tablespoons lemon juice
1/4 cup Kalamata olives, pitted and halved	2 cloves garlic, minced
	Salt and pepper to taste
2 tablespoons capers	2 tablespoons olive oil

1. Preheat the oven to 425°F (220°C).

2. Season chicken breast fillets with salt, pepper, and dried oregano. Heat olive oil in an oven-safe skillet over medium-high heat.

3. Sear the chicken breast fillets on both sides until golden brown.

4. Transfer the skillet to the preheated oven and roast for about 15-20 minutes, or until the chicken is cooked through.

5. In a separate bowl, combine pitted Kalamata olives, capers, minced garlic, lemon zest, and a drizzle of olive oil.

6. Remove the chicken from the oven and top each fillet with the olive and caper mixture.

7. Return the skillet to the oven for an additional 5 minutes to allow the flavors to meld.

Nutritional information per serving:

Kcal	Carbs	Protein	Fat	Sugar	Fiber
210	3g	22g	13g	1g	1g

DAY 3

15'   2

Ingredients:

1 cup rolled oats	1/4 teaspoon garlic
2 cups water	powder
1/2 teaspoon salt	1/4 teaspoon dried
1/4 teaspoon black	thyme
pepper	1/4 teaspoon dried
2 tablespoons chopped	oregano
fresh parsley	1/4 cup grated
	Parmesan cheese

1. In a saucepan, bring water or milk to a boil.

2. Stir in rolled oats, salt, and your choice of savory seasonings such as garlic powder, dried herbs, or grated Parmesan cheese.

3. Cook the oatmeal according to the package instructions until thick and creamy.

4. After the oatmeal has finished cooking, top it

with sautéed spinach, mushrooms, and cherry tomatoes. Add some cheese and fresh herbs as a garnish, if preferred.

Nutritional information per serving:

Kcal	Carbs	Protein	Fat	Sugar	Fiber
117	17g	5g	3g	1g	3g

25'   2

Ingredients:

1 cup bulgur wheat	¼ cup chopped fresh
2 cups water	mint
2 roasted red bell	2 tablespoons lemon
peppers, diced	juice
½ cup chopped fresh	2 tablespoons olive oil
parsley	Salt and pepper to
	taste

1. In a saucepan, heat olive oil over medium heat.

2. Add chopped onion and cook until translucent.

3. Stir in the bulgur and cook for a few minutes until lightly toasted.

4. Pour vegetable or chicken broth into the saucepan and bring it to a boil.

5. Reduce the heat to low, cover the saucepan, and simmer for about 15-20 minutes, or until the bulgur is tender and the liquid is absorbed.

6. Meanwhile, roast red bell peppers in the oven until the skin is charred.

7. Remove the peppers from the oven, let them cool slightly, then peel off the charred skin and slice them into strips.

8. Once the bulgur is cooked, fluff it with a fork and stir in the roasted red bell pepper strips.

9. Add salt, pepper and a squeeze of lemon juice.

Nutritional information per serving:

Kcal	Carbs	Protein	Fat	Sugar	Fiber
200	8g	5g	8g	2g	5g

Dinner: Simple and Easy Turkey Breast Fillet Wraps

 20'   2

Ingredients:

4 turkey breast fillets
4 whole wheat tortillas
1 cup mixed salad greens
1/2 cup sliced cucumber

1/2 cup sliced cherry tomatoes
1/4 cup Greek yogurt
2 tablespoons lemon juice
Salt and pepper to taste

1. Season turkey breast fillets with salt, pepper, and your choice of dried herbs.

2. Heat olive oil in a skillet over medium-high heat.

3. Cook the turkey breast fillets for about 4-5 minutes on each side until cooked through and nicely browned.

4. Remove the turkey from the skillet and let it rest for a few minutes.

5. Slice the turkey breast fillets into thin strips.

6. Spread a layer of hummus or Greek yogurt onto a whole wheat tortilla.

7. Place the sliced turkey, along with your choice of fresh vegetables like lettuce, tomatoes, cucumbers, and shredded carrots, onto the tortilla.

8. Roll the tortilla tightly to form a wrap.

9. Cut the wrap in half and secure with toothpicks if necessary.

Nutritional information per serving:

Kcal	Carbs	Protein	Fat	Sugar	Fiber
340	22g	45g	9g	3g	4g

DAY 4

Breakfast: Avocado Tomato and Egg

 15' 2

Ingredients:

2 ripe avocados	4 eggs
2 tomatoes, sliced	Salt and pepper to taste

1. Slice a ripe avocado in half, remove the pit, and scoop out the flesh into a bowl.

2. Mash the avocado with a fork until it reaches your desired consistency.

3. Toast a slice of whole-grain bread. Spread the mashed avocado on the toast. Top the avocado toast with sliced tomatoes.

4. In a separate skillet, fry an egg to your liking (e.g., sunny-side-up, over-easy, or scrambled).

5. Place the cooked egg on top of the avocado and tomato.

Nutritional information per serving:

Kcal	Carbs	Protein	Fat	Sugar	Fiber
162	8g	7g	13g	2g	5g

Lunch: Chickpea and Grape Salad

 10' 2

Ingredients:

2 cups cooked chickpeas	1/4 cup chopped fresh mint
1 cup halved grapes	2 tablespoons lemon juice
1/2 cup diced cucumber	2 tablespoons olive oil
1/4 cup chopped fresh parsley	Salt and pepper to taste

1. In a large mixing bowl, combine cooked chickpeas, halved grapes, chopped cucumber, diced red onion and crumbled feta cheese.

2. In a separate small bowl, whisk together olive oil, lemon juice, minced garlic, dried oregano, salt, and pepper to make the dressing.

3. Drizzle the dressing over the combination of grapes and chickpeas. All the ingredients should be well mixed with the dressing. If necessary, taste and adjust the seasoning.

4. Give the salad some time to rest so the flavors may mingle. Add some finely chopped fresh herbs just before serving.

Nutritional information per serving:

Kcal	Carbs	Protein	Fat	Sugar	Fiber
250	8g	11g	10g	10g	9g

Dinner: Mango and Coconut Frozen Pie

 10' 2

Ingredients:

2 ripe mangoes, peeled and diced	2 tablespoons lime juice
1 cup coconut milk	1/2 cup shredded coconut
1/4 cup honey	

1. Pulse the Graham crackers into tiny crumbs in a food processor. Add the melted butter to the crumbs after moving them to a mixing bowl.

2. To create the crust, press the crumbs mixture firmly into the bottom of a pie plate. Combine coconut milk, lime juice, and sweetened condensed milk in a separate mixing dish.

3. Stir until smooth and well blended. Fill the pie crust with the ingredients. Mango slices should be placed on top of the filling.

4. Put the pie in the freezer for at least 4 hours, or until it's solid. A few minutes before serving, take the pie out of the freezer to give it time to soften.

Nutritional information per serving:

Kcal	Carbs	Protein	Fat	Sugar	Fiber
373	42g	4g	24g	36g	5g

Breakfast: Baked Eggs with Cottage Cheese

  20' 2

Ingredients:

4 eggs	2 tablespoons
1 cup cottage cheese	chopped fresh chives
1/4 cup grated	Salt and pepper to
Parmesan cheese	taste

1. Preheat the oven to 375°F (190°C).

2. Grease individual ramekins or a baking dish with cooking spray or butter. Crack one or two eggs into each ramekin or spread them evenly in the baking dish.

3. Spoon cottage cheese on top of the eggs, ensuring each egg is covered. Season with salt, pepper, and your choice of herbs or spices.

4. Place the ramekins or baking dish in the preheated oven and bake for about 12-15 minutes.

Nutritional information per serving:

Kcal	Carbs	Protein	Fat	Sugar	Fiber
140	3g	14g	8g	2g	1g

Lunch: Tomato Basil Pasta

 20' 2

Ingredients:

6 ounces whole wheat pasta	1/4 cup chopped fresh basil
3 cloves garlic, minced	Salt and pepper to
4 cups cherry tomatoes, halved	taste
	2 tablespoons olive oil

1. Turn on the fire under the pot and wait for the water to boil. Add the salt and your favorite pasta, and cook according to the package instructions until al dente.

2. While the pasta is cooking, heat olive oil in a skillet over medium heat. Add minced garlic and sauté for a minute until fragrant.

3. Add diced tomatoes and cook for about 5 minutes until softened. Season with salt, pepper, and dried basil or fresh basil leaves.

4. Reduce the heat to low and simmer the tomato sauce for another 5 minutes. Drain the cooked pasta and add it to the skillet with the tomato sauce.

5. Toss the pasta with the sauce until well coated. Remove from the heat and let it sit for a few minutes to allow the flavors to meld together.

Nutritional information per serving:

Kcal	Carbs	Protein	Fat	Sugar	Fiber
290	48g	10g	10g	6g	8g

Dinner: Baked Lamb Chops

 25' 2

Ingredients

4 lamb chops	1 teaspoon dried
2 tablespoons olive oil	rosemary
2 cloves garlic, minced	Salt and pepper to taste

1. Preheat the oven to 400°F (200°C). Season lamb chops with salt, pepper, dried rosemary, and minced garlic, pressing the seasonings onto the meat.

2. In a skillet that is oven-safe, heat the olive oil over medium-high heat. The lamb chops should be browned after 2 minutes on each side of the pan.

3. Transfer the skillet to the preheated oven and bake for 10-12 minutes for medium-rare, or adjust the cooking time according to your preference.

4. Remove the pan from oven and let rest for 5 min

Nutritional information per serving:

Kcal	Carbs	Protein	Fat	Sugar	Fiber
300	1g	18g	25g	0g	1g

DAY 6

Breakfast: Crustless Tiropita	**Lunch:** Ritzy Veggie Chili

  25' 2

 30' 2

Breakfast: Crustless Tiropita

Ingredients:

1 cup feta cheese, crumbled	1/4 cup chopped fresh dill
1 cup ricotta cheese	Salt and pepper to taste
4 eggs	

1. Preheat the oven to 375°F (190°C) and grease a baking dish with cooking spray or butter.

2. In a mixing bowl, combine crumbled feta cheese, cottage cheese, grated Parmesan cheese, beaten eggs, chopped fresh parsley, and a pinch of black pepper.

3. Stir the mixture until well combined and pour it into the prepared baking dish.

4. Smooth the top with a spatula, and sprinkle additional grated Parmesan cheese on top.

5. Bake in the preheated oven for 25-30 minutes, or until the top is golden brown and the filling is set.

6. Remove it from the oven and let it cool for a few minutes before slicing into squares or wedges.

Nutritional information per serving:

Kcal	Carbs	Protein	Fat	Sugar	Fiber
250	6g	16g	20g	1g	0g

Lunch: Ritzy Veggie Chili

Ingredients:

1 tablespoon olive oil	1 can (5 ounces) kidney beans, drained and rinsed
1 onion, chopped	
2 cloves garlic, minced	1 can (5 ounces) diced tomatoes
1 bell pepper, diced	
1 zucchini, diced	1 cup vegetable broth
1 can (5 ounces) black beans, drained and rinsed	1 tablespoon chili powder
	Salt and pepper to taste

1. In a big saucepan or Dutch oven, heat the olive oil over medium heat.

2. Add bell peppers, minced garlic, and diced onions to the saucepan.

3. Sauté the veggies for about 5 minutes, or until they are tender.

4. Fill the pot with diced tomatoes, kidney beans that have been washed and drained, black beans that have also been rinsed and drained, corn, cumin, paprika, salt, and pepper. Stir everything together thoroughly.

5. Bring the mixture to a boil, then lower the heat to a simmer, stirring regularly, for 20 to 25 minutes. When necessary, taste and adjust the spices

Nutritional information per serving:

Kcal	Carbs	Protein	Fat	Sugar	Fiber
215	30g	10g	6g	5g	10g

Dinner: Pecan and Carrot Cake

 35' 2

Ingredients:

2 cups grated carrots
1 cup pecans, chopped
1 cup whole wheat flour
1/2 cup almond flour
1/2 cup coconut sugar

1/4 cup melted coconut oil
4 eggs
1 teaspoon baking powder
1 teaspoon cinnamon
1/2 teaspoon nutmeg
1/4 teaspoon salt

1. Preheat the oven to 350°F (175°C) and grease a cake pan with cooking spray or butter.

2. In a mixing bowl, combine all-purpose flour, whole wheat flour, baking powder, baking soda, ground cinnamon, and a pinch of salt.

3. In a separate bowl, whisk together granulated sugar, brown sugar, vegetable oil, eggs, and vanilla extract until well combined.

4. Gradually add the dry ingredients to the wet ingredients and mix until just combined.

5. Fold in shredded carrots, chopped pecans, and raisins.

6. Pour the batter into the prepared cake pan and smooth the top with a spatula.

7. Bake in the preheated oven for about 35-40 minutes, or until a toothpick inserted into the center comes out clean.

8. Remove the cake from the oven and let it cool in the pan for 10 minutes before transferring it to a wire rack to cool completely.

9. Once the cake has cooled, you can optionally frost it with cream cheese frosting or simply dust it with powdered sugar.

10. Slice and serve the moist and nutty pecan and carrot cake as a delightful dessert.

Nutritional information per serving:

Kcal	Carbs	Protein	Fat	Sugar	Fiber
660	60g	14g	44g	30g	10g

DAY 7

Breakfast: Mediterranean Vegetable Omelet	**Lunch:** Caprese Fusilli

 15'   2   20'   2

Ingredients:

4 large eggs	¼ cup diced red onions
¼ cup diced bell peppers	¼ cup crumbled feta cheese
¼ cup diced tomatoes	1 tablespoon olive oil
¼ cup chopped spinach	Salt and pepper to taste

1. Beat the eggs and season them with salt and pepper in a bowl.

2. In a nonstick skillet over medium heat, warm the olive oil.

3. Add the spinach, red onions, bell peppers, tomatoes, and spinach to the skillet. 1-2 minutes of sautéing is sufficient to mildly tenderize the veggies.

4. Pour the beaten eggs on top of the skillet's veggies. Cook until the edges are firm, about a few minutes.

5. Evenly cover the omelet with feta cheese.

6. To melt the cheese, carefully flip the omelet in half and cook for one more minute.

7. Slide the omelet onto a plate and serve hot.

Nutritional Information (per serving):

Kcal	Carbs	Protein	Fat	Sugar	Fiber
136	2g	8g	10g	1g	1g

Ingredients:

6 ounces whole wheat fusilli pasta	1/2 cup fresh basil leaves, torn
2 cups cherry tomatoes, halved	2 tablespoons balsamic glaze
6 ounces fresh mozzarella cheese, diced	Salt and pepper to taste

1. Turn on the fire under the pot and wait for the water to boil. Add the salt and fusilli, and cook according to the package instructions until al dente.

2. While the pasta is cooking. In a mixing bowl, combine cherry tomatoes (halved), mozzarella cheese balls (halved), fresh basil leaves (torn), and cooked fusilli pasta.

3. Drizzle extra-virgin olive oil over the pasta mixture and season with salt and pepper to taste.

4. Toss all the ingredients gently to combine and coat with the dressing.

5. Let the flavors meld together by refrigerating the caprese fusilli for at least 30 minutes.

Nutritional information per serving:

Kcal	Carbs	Protein	Fat	Sugar	Fiber
400	50g	21g	14g	7g	6g

Dinner: Zucchini and Artichokes Bowl with Farro

 25' 2

Ingredients:

1 cup farro
2 zucchinis, sliced
1 can (7 ounces) artichoke hearts, drained and quartered

1/4 cup sun-dried tomatoes, chopped
2 cloves garlic, minced
2 tablespoons olive oil
Juice of 1 lemon
Salt and pepper to taste

1. Cook farro according to package instructions until tender.

2. Heat olive oil in a large skillet over medium heat.

3. Add sliced zucchini, drained and quartered artichoke hearts, minced garlic, and a pinch of red pepper flakes to the skillet.

4. Sauté for about 5-7 minutes until the zucchini is tender.

5. Stir in cooked farro and season with salt, pepper, and dried herbs like oregano or basil.

6. Cook for an additional 2-3 minutes to allow the flavors to blend.

7. Remove from heat and garnish with chopped fresh parsley or basil.

8. Serve the flavorful zucchini and artichokes bowl with farro as a wholesome and satisfying dinner.

Nutritional information per serving:

Kcal	Carbs	Protein	Fat	Sugar	Fiber
262	41g	7g	8g	6g	6g

DAY 8

Breakfast: Berry and Nut Parfait

 10'   2

Ingredients:

1 cup Greek yogurt
1 cup mixed berries
(strawberries,
blueberries,
raspberries)
¼ cup granola

2 tablespoons
chopped nuts
(almonds, walnuts, or
pistachios)
1 tablespoon honey

1. In a glass or jar, layer Greek yogurt, mixed berries (such as strawberries, blueberries, and raspberries), and a handful of chopped nuts (such as almonds, walnuts, or pistachios).

2. Repeat the layers until the glass or jar is filled.

3. Drizzle a small amount of honey or maple syrup over the top for added sweetness, if desired.

4. Garnish with a sprig of fresh mint.

5. Enjoy this delicious and nutritious berry and nut parfait for breakfast.

Nutritional information per serving:

Kcal	Carbs	Protein	Fat	Sugar	Fiber
136	15g	6g	6g	10g	2g

Lunch: Walnut and Ricotta Spaghetti

 20'   2

Ingredients:

6 ounces whole wheat
spaghetti
1 cup ricotta cheese
1/2 cup chopped
walnuts
2 tablespoons extra
virgin olive oil

2 cloves garlic,
minced
1/4 cup chopped fresh
parsley
Salt and pepper to
taste

1. Turn on the fire under the pot and wait for the water to boil. Add the salt and the spaghetti, and cook according to the package instructions until al dente.

2. Meanwhile, heat olive oil in a skillet over medium heat.

3. Add minced garlic and cook until fragrant, about 1 minute.

4. Add crushed walnuts to the skillet and toast them for a few minutes until lightly browned.

5. In a separate bowl, combine ricotta cheese, lemon zest, lemon juice, and a pinch of salt and pepper.

6. Drain the cooked spaghetti and transfer it to the skillet with the toasted walnuts.

7. Add the ricotta mixture to the skillet and toss well to coat the pasta evenly. Adjust the seasoning if needed

Nutritional information per serving:

Kcal	Carbs	Protein	Fat	Sugar	Fiber
465	48g	15g	25g	2g	7g

Dinner: Garlicky Zucchini Cubes with Mint

 15'   *2*

Ingredients:

4 zucchinis, cut into cubes	Juice of 1 lemon
3 cloves garlic, minced	2 tablespoons chopped fresh mint
2 tablespoons olive oil	Salt and pepper to taste

1. In a big pan over medium heat, warm the olive oil.

2. Add diced zucchini and minced garlic to the skillet.

3. Sauté until the zucchini is tender and lightly golden brown.

4. Season with salt, pepper, and a pinch of red pepper flakes for some heat.

5. Remove from the heat and sprinkle freshly chopped mint leaves over the zucchini cubes.

6. Toss gently to incorporate the mint flavor.

7. Transfer to a serving dish and drizzle with a squeeze of fresh lemon juice.

8. Serve the garlicky zucchini cubes with mint as a flavorful and healthy dinner option.

Nutritional information per serving:

Kcal	Carbs	Protein	Fat	Sugar	Fiber
101	8g	3g	7g	5g	2g

DAY 9

Breakfast: Kale and Apple Smoothie

 10' 2

Ingredients:

2 cups kale leaves, stems removed
1 apple, cored and chopped
1/2 banana

1/2 cup almond milk (or any other milk of your choice)
1 tablespoon honey or maple syrup
1/2 teaspoon ground cinnamon

1. In a blender, combine fresh kale leaves, chopped apple, Greek yogurt, almond milk, and a drizzle of honey.

2. Blend until creamy and smooth.

3. If necessary, change the consistency by adding additional almond milk.

4. Place the smoothie in a glass and top with a few apple slices or a sprinkle of cinnamon.

5. Enjoy this nutritious and refreshing kale and apple smoothie for breakfast

Nutritional information per serving:

Kcal	Carbs	Protein	Fat	Sugar	Fiber
77	18g	2g	1g	13g	3g

Lunch: Chard and Mushroom Risotto

 30' 2

Ingredients:

1 cup arborio rice
4 cups vegetable broth
2 tablespoons olive oil
1 onion, finely chopped
2 cloves garlic, minced

8 ounces mushrooms, sliced
4 cups chard leaves, chopped
¼ cup grated Parmesan cheese
Salt and pepper

1. In a large saucepan, heat olive oil over medium heat.

2. Add chopped onions and minced garlic to the pan and sauté until translucent.

3. Add sliced mushrooms and cook until they release their moisture and become tender.

4. Stir in Arborio rice and cook for a couple of minutes, allowing it to toast slightly.

5. Pour in vegetable broth a little at a time, stirring constantly until the liquid is absorbed.

6. Continue adding broth and stirring until the rice is cooked al dente and has a creamy consistency.

7. Meanwhile, blanch chard leaves in boiling water for a few minutes until wilted, then drain and chop.

8. Stir the chopped chard into the risotto along with the grated Parmesan cheese.

9. Season with salt, pepper, and a pinch of nutmeg for added flavor.

10. Remove from heat, cover, and let it rest for a few minutes before serving.

Nutritional information per serving:

Kcal	Carbs	Protein	Fat	Sugar	Fiber
300	48g	8g	9g	4g	2g

Dinner: Parsley-Dijon Chicken and Potatoes

 30' 2

Ingredients:

4 chicken breasts
4 cups baby potatoes, halved
2 tablespoons Dijon mustard

2 tablespoons chopped fresh parsley
2 tablespoons olive oil
Juice of 1 lemon
Salt and pepper to taste

1. Preheat the oven to 400°F (200°C).

2. In a small bowl, mix together minced garlic, chopped fresh parsley, Dijon mustard, olive oil, salt, and pepper.

3. Place chicken breasts and quartered potatoes in a baking dish.

4. Pour the parsley-Dijon mixture over the chicken and potatoes, making sure to coat them evenly.

5. Roast in the preheated oven for about 25-30 minutes, or until the chicken is cooked through and the potatoes are golden and crispy.

6. Remove it from the oven and let it rest for a few minutes.

7. Serve the flavorful parsley-Dijon chicken with potatoes for a satisfying dinner.

Nutritional information per serving:

Kcal	Carbs	Protein	Fat	Sugar	Fiber
576	25g	51g	30g	1g	2g

DAY 10

Breakfast: Calo Cinnamon Oatmeal

 15' 2

Ingredients:

1 cup rolled oats
2 cups water
½ cup almond milk
(or any other milk of
your choice)

1 tablespoon honey or
maple syrup
½ teaspoon ground
cinnamon
Optional toppings:
sliced bananas,
chopped nuts, raisins

1. In a saucepan, bring water to a boil.

2. Add rolled oats, ground cinnamon, and a pinch of salt to the boiling water.

3. Reduce heat to low and simmer for about 5 minutes, stirring occasionally.

4. Stir in a splash of milk (dairy or plant-based) to achieve your desired consistency.

5. Remove from heat and let it sit for a minute to thicken.

6. Transfer the oatmeal to a bowl and garnish with your favorite toppings, such as sliced bananas, chopped nuts, and a drizzle of honey.

7. Enjoy the comforting and nutritious Calo Cinnamon Oatmeal for breakfast.

Nutritional information per serving:

Kcal	Carbs	Protein	Fat	Sugar	Fiber
190	32g	5g	6g	11g	4g

Lunch: Pesto Pasta

 20' 2

Ingredients:

6 ounces whole wheat
pasta
2 cups fresh basil
leaves
1/2 cup grated
Parmesan cheese

2 cloves garlic
1/2 cup olive oil
Salt and pepper to
taste
1/4 cup pine nuts

1. Turn on the fire under the pot and wait for the water to boil. Add the salt and the pasta, and cook according to the package instructions until al dente.

2. Meanwhile, prepare the pesto sauce by blending fresh basil leaves, pine nuts, grated Parmesan cheese, minced garlic, and olive oil in a food processor or blender until smooth.

3. Drain the cooked pasta and return it to the pot.

4. Add the pesto sauce to the pasta and toss until well coated.

5. If desired, you can also add cooked cherry tomatoes or sautéed vegetables for extra flavor and nutrition.

6. Season with salt and pepper to taste.

Note: Remember that pesto must be put in the pot with the heat off; it should not be cooked

Nutritional information per serving:

Kcal	Carbs	Protein	Fat	Sugar	Fiber
550	45g	13g	37g	1g	6g

Dinner: Cauliflower Hash with Carrots

 20' 2

Ingredients:

1 head cauliflower, cut into florets
2 carrots, diced
1 onion, diced
2 cloves garlic, minced

2 tablespoons olive oil
1 teaspoon smoked paprika
Salt and pepper to taste
Optional toppings: fresh herbs, such as parsley or chives

1. Preheat the oven to 425°F (220°C).

2. Chop cauliflower into small florets and dice carrots into small pieces.

3. In a large mixing bowl, combine cauliflower florets, diced carrots, minced garlic, dried thyme, paprika, salt, and pepper.

4. Drizzle olive oil over the vegetables and toss to coat them evenly with the seasonings.

5. Spread the seasoned vegetables on a baking sheet in a single layer.

6. Roast in the preheated oven for about 25-30 minutes, or until the cauliflower and carrots are tender and slightly browned.

7. Remove from the oven and serve the flavorful cauliflower hash as a nutritious and delicious dinner option.

Nutritional information per serving:

Kcal	Carbs	Protein	Fat	Sugar	Fiber
105	9g	2g	8g	4g	3g

DAY 11

10'   2   10'   30'   2

Ingredients:

1 cup Greek yogurt
1 cup mixed fresh fruits (such as berries, sliced banana, and diced mango)

2 tablespoons honey or maple syrup
Optional toppings: granola, nuts, or shredded coconut

1. Choose your favorite fruits, such as berries, sliced banana, diced mango, or chopped apples.

2. In a bowl, spoon some plain Greek yogurt or your preferred yogurt variety.

3. Add the assortment of fruits on top of the yogurt.

4. Optional: Sprinkle with a drizzle of honey or a sprinkle of granola for added sweetness and crunch.

5. Mix the fruits and yogurt together gently.

6. Enjoy the refreshing and nutritious fruit yogurt for breakfast.

Nutritional information per serving:

Kcal	Carbs	Protein	Fat	Sugar	Fiber
250	27g	20g	9g	20g	5g

Ingredients:

2 tablespoons olive oil
1 medium onion, finely chopped
2 cloves garlic, minced
8 ounces mushrooms (such as cremini or button mushrooms), sliced
1 cup Arborio rice

4 cups vegetable or chicken broth
1/2 cup white wine (optional)
1/2 cup grated Parmesan cheese
2 tablespoons butter
Salt and pepper to taste
Fresh parsley,

1. In a big, deep pot or skillet over medium heat, warm the olive oil. Cook for two to three minutes, or until the onion is translucent, after adding the minced garlic and onion.

2. Include the mushroom slices in the pan and boil for 5 minutes, or until the mushrooms begin to release moisture and become brown.

3. Add the Arborio rice and stir continuously for a further 2 minutes of cooking.

4. Add the white wine, if using, and boil the rice, stirring regularly, until the liquid has almost been absorbed.

5. Start adding the broth, stirring regularly, approximately 1/2 cup at a time. Before adding extra broth, let the rice absorb the previous addition. Continue doing this until the risotto is creamy and the rice is al dente. It should just take 20 to 25 minutes to do this.

6. Once the butter has melted, add it along with the Parmesan cheese. To taste, add salt

7. Turn off the heat and allow the risotto cool for a while so it can thicken.

Nutritional Information (per serving):

Kcal	Carbs	Protein	Fat	Sugar	Fiber

367   46g   9g   15g   3g   1g

Dinner: Lemon Garlic Shrimp Skewers

 10'   10'   ⊗ 2

Ingredients:

10/12 ounces large
shrimp, peeled and
deveined
2 tablespoons olive oil
2 cloves garlic, minced
Zest and juice of 1
lemon

1 teaspoon dried
oregano
Salt and pepper to
taste
Skewers (if using
wooden skewers, soak
them in water for 30
minutes before
grilling)

1. To create the marinade, mix the olive oil, minced garlic, lemon juice, lemon zest, dried oregano, salt, and pepper in a bowl.

2. Include the peeled and deveined shrimp in the marinade, tossing to thoroughly distribute the coating. Give the shrimp about 10 minutes to marinate.

3. Set the grill's temperature to medium-high. The marinated shrimp are threaded onto skewers.

4. Grill the shrimp for two to three minutes on each side, or until they are opaque and fully cooked.

5. Take the food off the grill and serve it right away with your choice of sides or a crisp salad.

Nutritional Information (per serving):

Kcal	Carbs	Protein	Fat	Sugar	Fiber
141	2g	15g	8g	0.25g	1g

DAY 12

Breakfast: Avocado Toast with Goat Cheese

 10' 2

Ingredients:

2 slices whole grain bread

1 ripe avocado

2 ounces goat cheese

1 tablespoon lemon juice

Salt and pepper to taste

1. Toast a slice of whole-grain bread until golden and crispy.

2. While the bread is toasting, prepare the avocado spread by mashing a ripe avocado in a bowl.

3. Season the mashed avocado with salt, pepper, and a squeeze of fresh lemon juice for added flavor.

4. Spread the mashed avocado mixture onto the toasted bread.

5. Crumble some goat cheese over the avocado spread.

6. Optional: Top with a sprinkle of red pepper flakes or a drizzle of honey for a hint of spice or sweetness.

7. Serve the avocado toast as a delicious and nutritious breakfast.

Nutritional information per serving:

Kcal	Carbs	Protein	Fat	Sugar	Fiber
117	8g	5g	7g	2g	3g

Lunch: Garlic Shrimp Fettuccine

 20' 2

Ingredients:

6 ounces fettuccine pasta

12 ounces shrimp, peeled and deveined

4 cloves garlic, minced

2 tablespoons olive oil

¼ cup white wine

¼ cup fresh parsley, chopped

Salt and pepper to taste

1. Turn on the fire under the pot and wait for the water to boil. Add the salt and the fettuccine, and cook according to the package instructions until al dente.

2. While the pasta is cooking, heat olive oil in a large skillet over medium heat.

3. Add minced garlic to the skillet and sauté until fragrant.

4. Add peeled and deveined shrimp to the skillet and cook until pink and cooked through.

5. Season the shrimp with salt, pepper, and red pepper flakes for some heat.

6. Drain the cooked pasta and combine it with the shrimp in the skillet.

7. Toss the pasta and shrimp together, allowing them to combine and heat through.

8. Squeeze fresh lemon juice over the pasta for a burst of citrus flavor.

Nutritional information per serving:

Kcal	Carbs	Protein	Fat	Sugar	Fiber
342	31g	30g	10g	0g	2g

Dinner: Sweet Potato and Tomato Curry

 30' 2

Ingredients:

2 medium sweet potatoes, peeled and cubed
1 can diced tomatoes
1 can coconut milk
1 onion, chopped
2 cloves garlic, minced

1 tablespoon curry powder
1 teaspoon ground turmeric
1 teaspoon ground cumin
Salt and pepper to taste

1. Heat oil in a large saucepan over medium heat.

2. Add diced onion and minced garlic to the saucepan and sauté until the onion is translucent.

3. Stir in curry powder, ground cumin, ground coriander, and turmeric powder.

4. Add diced sweet potatoes, diced tomatoes, and vegetable broth to the saucepan.

5. Bring the mixture to a boil, then reduce the heat and let it simmer until the sweet potatoes are tender.

6. Add coconut milk and stir well to combine.

7. Season with salt and pepper to taste.

8. Simmer the curry for a few more minutes to allow the flavors to meld together.

9. Optional: Garnish with chopped fresh cilantro or a squeeze of lime juice.

10. Serve the sweet potato and tomato curry over steamed rice or with naan bread for a delicious and hearty dinner.

Nutritional information per serving:

Kcal	Carbs	Protein	Fat	Sugar	Fiber
295	28g	5g	20g	5g	5g

DAY 13

Breakfast: Banana-Blueberry Breakfast Cookies

 20' 2

Ingredients:

2 ripe bananas, mashed
1 cup rolled oats
1/2 cup almond butter
1/4 cup honey

1/4 cup dried blueberries
1/4 cup chopped walnuts
1/2 teaspoon cinnamon

1. Set a baking sheet on your oven's 350°F (175°C) rack and preheat the oven.

2. Smoothly mash two ripe bananas in a mixing dish.

3. To the bowl of mashed bananas, add rolled oats, almond flour, honey, cinnamon, and vanilla extract.

4. Stir in dried blueberries and chopped nuts of your choice (such as walnuts or almonds).

5. Mix all the ingredients until well combined, and the mixture forms a sticky dough.

6. Take scoops of the dough and shape them into cookies, placing them on the prepared baking sheet.

7. Flatten each cookie slightly with the back of a spoon.

8. Bake the cookies in the preheated oven for 12-15 minutes, or until they are lightly golden around the edges.

9. Remove the cookies from the oven and let them cool before serving.

Nutritional information per serving (2 cookies):

Kcal	Carbs	Protein	Fat	Sugar	Fiber
486	62g	12g	25g	33g	8g

Lunch: Lentil Risotto

 10' 30' 2

Ingredients:

1 cup green lentils
2 cups vegetable broth
1 tablespoon olive oil
1 onion, chopped
2 cloves garlic, minced

1 cup Arborio rice
1/4 cup white wine
1/2 cup grated Parmesan cheese
Salt and pepper to taste

1. Heat the olive oil in a big pot over medium heat.

2. Add chopped onion and minced garlic to the pan and cook, stirring occasionally, until the onion is translucent and tender.

3. Add the Arborio rice and stir. Cook for a few minutes, until the rice is thoroughly covered in oil.

4. Add a small amount of vegetable broth at a time, stirring continuously until the liquid is completely absorbed.

5. Keep doing this until the rice is creamy and al dente, adding liquid as you go and tossing.

6. In a separate skillet, heat a little olive oil and sauté diced vegetables of your choice (such as carrots, bell peppers, and zucchini) until tender.

7. Add the cooked vegetables to the risotto and stir to combine.

8. Stir in cooked lentils and season with salt, pepper, and herbs of your choice.

Nutritional information per serving:

Kcal	Carbs	Protein	Fat	Sugar	Fiber
443	71g	20g	8g	4g	15g

Dinner: Macadamia Pork

 25'   ⊗ 2

Ingredients:

4 boneless pork chops	1 tablespoon honey
1/2 cup macadamia nuts, crushed	1/4 teaspoon salt
2 tablespoons Dijon mustard	1/4 teaspoon black pepper

1. Preheat your oven to 375°F (190°C) and lightly grease a baking dish.

2. In a small bowl, mix together crushed macadamia nuts, bread crumbs, grated Parmesan cheese, dried herbs (such as thyme or rosemary), and a pinch of salt and pepper.

3. Season pork chops with salt and pepper on both sides.

4. Dip each pork chop into beaten eggs, allowing any excess to drip off.

5. Press both sides of the pork chop into the macadamia nut mixture, coating it well.

6. Place the coated pork chops in the prepared baking dish.

7. Bake in the preheated oven for 20-25 minutes, or until the pork is cooked through and the crust is golden brown.

8. Remove the pork chops from the oven and let them rest for a few minutes before serving.

Nutritional information per serving:

Kcal	Carbs	Protein	Fat	Sugar	Fiber
395	7g	32g	26g	5g	2g

DAY 14

Breakfast: Blackberry-Yogurt Green Smoothie	**Lunch:** Cheesy Tomato Linguine

 10' 2   20' 2

Ingredients:

1 cup blackberries	1 cup spinach
½ cup plain Greek yogurt	½ cup almond milk
1 banana	1 tablespoon honey

1. In a blender, combine fresh blackberries, plain Greek yogurt, baby spinach leaves, almond milk, and a drizzle of honey.

2. Combine and blend the items until they are smooth.

3. If preferred, add ice cubes to the blender and reblend the smoothie until it has the consistency you want.

4. Pour a glass with the smoothie inside, then serve right away.

Nutritional information per serving:

Kcal	Carbs	Protein	Fat	Sugar	Fiber
102	18g	4g	3g	13g	3g

Ingredients:

6 ounces linguine pasta	1/4 teaspoon red pepper flakes
2 tablespoons olive oil	1/2 cup grated Parmesan cheese
3 cloves garlic, minced	Salt and pepper to taste
1 can (10 ounces) diced tomato	

1. Turn on the fire under the pot and wait for the water to boil. Add the salt and the linguine, and cook according to the package instructions until al dente.

2. While the pasta is cooking. In a large skillet, heat olive oil over medium heat.

Add minced garlic and cook until fragrant, about 1 minute.

3. Stir in the diced tomatoes and cook for a few minutes until the tomatoes soften.

4. Season with salt, pepper, and dried basil or Italian seasoning to taste.

5. Reduce the heat to low and add the cooked linguine to the skillet.

6. Toss the linguine with the tomato mixture until well coated.

7. Sprinkle grated Parmesan cheese and shredded mozzarella cheese over the linguine.

8. Cover the skillet with a lid and let the cheese melt for a few minutes.

Nutritional information per serving:

Kcal	Carbs	Protein	Fat	Sugar	Fiber
334	47g	12g	11g	2g	2g

Dinner: Glazed Mushroom and Vegetable Fajitas

 25' 2

Ingredients:

2 tablespoons olive oil
1 onion, sliced
2 bell peppers, sliced
8 ounces mushrooms, sliced
2 cloves garlic, minced
2 tablespoons soy sauce

1 tablespoon honey
1 teaspoon ground cumin
1/2 teaspoon smoked paprika
Salt and pepper to taste
Whole wheat tortillas, for serving

1. In a large skillet, heat olive oil over medium-high heat.

2. Add sliced bell peppers, sliced onions, and sliced mushrooms to the skillet.

3. Sauté the vegetables until they are tender-crisp and slightly caramelized.

4. In a small bowl, whisk together soy sauce, honey, lime juice, minced garlic, and chili powder.

5. Pour the sauce over the sautéed vegetables and stir well to coat.

6. Continue cooking for a few more minutes until the vegetables are coated in the glaze and the sauce has thickened slightly.

7. Warm tortillas in a separate skillet or oven.

8. Spoon the glazed mushroom and vegetable mixture onto the warm tortillas.

9. Serve the fajitas with additional toppings such as sliced avocado, salsa, and sour cream, if desired.

Nutritional information per serving:

Kcal	Carbs	Protein	Fat	Sugar	Fiber
124	13g	4g	8g	4g	3g

DAY 15

Breakfast: Spinach Cheese Pie

 30'   2

Ingredients:

1 tablespoon olive oil
1 onion, chopped
2 cloves garlic, minced
8 ounces fresh spinach

4 large eggs
1 cup ricotta cheese
1/2 cup feta cheese, crumbled
Salt and pepper to taste
1 prepared pie crust

1. Preheat your oven to the temperature specified on the pie crust package.

2. In a large skillet, heat olive oil over medium heat.

3. Add chopped spinach and minced garlic to the skillet and sauté until the spinach is wilted and the garlic is fragrant.

4. Remove the skillet from the heat and let the spinach cool slightly.

5. In a mixing bowl, combine beaten eggs, crumbled feta cheese, grated Parmesan cheese, and the sautéed spinach mixture.

6. Line a pie dish with a pre-made pie crust.

7. Pour the spinach and cheese mixture into the pie crust and spread it evenly.

8. Place the pie dish in the preheated oven and bake according to the pie crust package instructions, or until the crust is golden brown and the filling is set.

9. Remove the pie from the oven and let it cool

Nutritional information per serving:

Kcal	Carbs	Protein	Fat	Sugar	Fiber
530	40g	18g	34g	2g	3g

Lunch: Spaghetti Ragù Bolognese

 10'   30'   2

Ingredients:

6 ounces spaghetti
2 tablespoons olive oil
1 onion, chopped
2 cloves garlic, minced
8 ounces ground chicken
1 can (8 ounces) crushed tomatoes

1 tablespoon tomato paste
1 teaspoon dried basil
1 teaspoon dried oregano
Salt and pepper to taste

1. Heat the olive oil in a big pan over medium heat.

2. In a pan, combine chopped onions and minced garlic, and cook until the onions are transparent.

3. Add ground meat to the skillet and cook until browned, breaking it up into small pieces with a spatula.

4. Stir in tomato paste, crushed tomatoes, dried basil, dried oregano, salt, and pepper.

5. Reduce the heat to low and let the sauce simmer for about 20-30 minutes to allow the flavors to meld together.

6. Cook spaghetti according to the package instructions until al dente. Drain and put in the skillet with the sauce

7. Serve the spaghetti on individual plates or bowls. Top with other ragù Bolognese sauces if you like. Garnish with grated Parmesan cheese

Nutritional information per serving:

Kcal	Carbs	Protein	Fat	Sugar	Fiber
403	53g	20g	13g	8g	5g

Dinner: Spicy Tofu Tacos with Cherry Tomato Salsa

 20' 2

Ingredients:

1 block (10 ounces) firm tofu, drained and crumbled	Salt and pepper to taste
2 tablespoons olive oil	1 cup cherry tomatoes, halved
1 teaspoon chili powder	1/4 cup red onion, finely chopped
1/2 teaspoon cumin	1/4 cup fresh cilantro, chopped
1/2 teaspoon paprika	Juice of 1 lime
1/4 teaspoon cayenne pepper	Corn tortillas, for serving

1. Drain and press the tofu to remove excess moisture.

2. Cut tofu into small cubes or strips and season with your preferred taco seasoning or a combination of spices such as chili powder, cumin, paprika, garlic powder, and salt.

3. In a large skillet, heat oil over medium heat.

4. Add the seasoned tofu to the skillet and cook until crispy and golden brown on all sides.

5. Meanwhile, prepare the cherry tomato salsa by combining halved cherry tomatoes, diced red onion, chopped cilantro, lime juice, minced jalapeno (adjust amount according to desired spice level), salt, and pepper in a bowl. Mix well.

6. Warm corn tortillas in a separate skillet or oven.

7. Assemble the tacos by placing a generous amount of the crispy tofu in each tortilla.

8. Top with the cherry tomato salsa and any additional toppings such as avocado slices, shredded lettuce, and hot sauce.

9. Serve the spicy tofu tacos immediately, and enjoy!

Nutritional information per serving:

Kcal	Carbs	Protein	Fat	Sugar	Fiber
164	5g	12g	12g	2g	2g

DAY 16

Breakfast: Baked Ricotta with Honey Pears

 25' 2

Ingredients:

2 pears, peeled, cored, and sliced
1 tablespoon honey
1 cup ricotta cheese
1 tablespoon lemon zest
1 tablespoon fresh thyme leaves

1. Preheat your oven to a moderate temperature.

2. Slice pears into thin wedges and remove the core and seeds.

3. In a small baking dish, place the pear slices in a single layer.

4. Drizzle the pears with honey and sprinkle them with cinnamon.

5. Bake in the preheated oven for about 15-20 minutes, or until the pears are soft and slightly caramelized.

6. While the pears are baking, place the ricotta cheese in a separate bowl and mix until smooth.

7. Remove the pears from the oven and let them cool slightly.

8. Serve a dollop of ricotta cheese on a plate and top with the baked pears.

9. Drizzle with additional honey if desired.

Nutritional information per serving:

Kcal	Carbs	Protein	Fat	Sugar	Fiber
150	20g	5g	7g	6g	3g

Lunch: Black Bean Chili with Mangoes

 30' 2

Ingredients:

1 tablespoon olive oil
1 onion, chopped
2 cloves garlic, minced
1 red bell pepper, chopped
1 jalapeño pepper, seeded and minced
Salt and pepper to taste
1 mango, diced
2 teaspoons chili powder
1 teaspoon cumin
1 can (7 ounces) black beans, drained and rinsed
1 can (7 ounces) diced tomatoes
1 cup vegetable broth

1. Heat the olive oil in a big saucepan or Dutch oven over medium heat.

2. To the saucepan, add chopped bell peppers, diced onions, and minced garlic. Sauté until the veggies are soft

3. Add chili powder, cumin, paprika, and oregano to the pot and stir to coat the vegetables with the spices.

4. Pour in the vegetable broth and bring to a simmer. Add canned black beans (rinsed and drained), diced tomatoes (with juices), and diced mangoes to the pot.

5. Cover the pot and let the chili simmer for about 20-30 minutes to allow the flavors to meld together. Taste and adjust the seasoning if needed.

Nutritional information per serving:

Kcal	Carb	Protein	Fat	Sugar	Fiber
177	27g	7g	6g	7g	7g

Dinner: Roasted Tomato Panini

 20'   2

Ingredients:

4 ciabatta rolls	4 tablespoons pesto
4 large tomatoes, sliced	sauce
	1 tablespoon balsamic
4 ounces fresh mozzarella cheese, sliced	glaze

1. Turn on the oven to a high setting.

2. Place tomatoes on a baking pan after slicing them into thick slices.

3. Add salt and pepper and drizzle olive oil over the tomato slices.

4. Roast the tomatoes for 15 to 20 minutes in a preheated oven, or until they are tender and just beginning to caramelize.

5. While the tomatoes are roasting, prepare the panini bread by slicing it in half lengthwise.

6. Spread pesto sauce on one side of each bread slice.

7. Layer the roasted tomato slices, fresh mozzarella cheese slices, and fresh basil leaves on top of the pesto.

8. Close the panini sandwiches and lightly brush the outer sides of the bread with olive oil.

9. Heat a panini press or grill pan over medium heat.

10. Place the prepared panini sandwiches on the heated press or grill pan and cook until the bread is crispy and the cheese is melted, pressing down gently with a spatula if using a grill pan.

11. Remove the panini from the press or grill pan and let them cool for a minute before slicing in half.

Nutritional information per serving:

Kcal	Carbs	Protein	Fat	Sugar	Fiber
381	50g	15g	14g	7g	4g

DAY 17

Breakfast: Pancakes with Berry Sauce

 20' 2

Ingredients:

1 cup all-purpose flour
2 tablespoons sugar
1 teaspoon baking powder
1/2 teaspoon baking soda
1/4 teaspoon salt
1 cup buttermilk

1 egg
2 tablespoons unsalted butter, melted
1 cup mixed berries (strawberries, blueberries, raspberri)
2 tablespoons maple syrup

1. Combine the flour, baking powder, sugar, and salt in a large mixing basin.

2. Combine the eggs, milk, and vanilla extract in another dish.

3. Add the wet ingredients in small amounts to the dry ingredients and whisk just until incorporated.

4. Lightly oil a nonstick skillet or griddle with butter or cooking spray before heating it over medium heat.

5. Pour about ¼ cup of the pancake batter onto the hot skillet for each pancake.

6. Cook the pancakes until surface bubbles appear, then turn them over and continue cooking the second side until golden.

7. Remove the cooked pancakes from the skillet and keep them warm.

8. In a small saucepan, combine fresh or frozen berries with a little water and cook over medium heat until the berries soften and release their juices.

9. Mash the berries with a fork or blend them until you have a smooth sauce.

Nutritional information per serving:

Kcal	Carbs	Protein	Fat	Sugar	Fiber
280	42g	7g	9g	18g	2g

Lunch: Italian Sautéed Cannellini Beans

 25' 2

Ingredients:

2 tablespoons olive oil
1 onion, diced
3 cloves garlic, minced
1 can (10 ounces) cannellini beans, drained and rinsed

1 can (10 ounces) diced tomatoes
1 teaspoon dried oregano
Salt and pepper to taste
Fresh basil leaves for garnish

1. Heat olive oil in a skillet over medium heat.

2. Add minced garlic and chopped onions to the skillet and sauté until the onions are translucent.

3. Add drained and rinsed canned cannellini beans to the skillet.

4. Season with salt, pepper, dried oregano, and red pepper flakes to taste.

5. Cook the beans, stirring occasionally, until they are heated through and start to slightly brown.

6. Add fresh chopped tomatoes and continue cooking for a few more minutes until the tomatoes soften.

7. Remove from heat and sprinkle with freshly chopped parsley.

8. Serve as a warm side dish or as a topping for toasted bread.

Nutritional information per serving:

Kcal	Carbs	Protein	Fat	Sugar	Fiber
233	26g	10g	8g	2g	11g

Dinner: Vegetable and Cheese Lavash Pizza

 25' 2

Ingredients:

2 whole wheat lavash bread	1 cup sliced zucchini
1 cup marinara sauce	1 cup sliced mushrooms
1 cup shredded mozzarella cheese	1/2 cup sliced red onions
1 cup sliced bell peppers (red, yellow, green)	1/2 teaspoon dried oregano
	Fresh basil leaves for garnish

1. Preheat your oven to a high temperature.

2. Place a lavash bread on a baking sheet lined with parchment paper.

3. Spread tomato sauce or pesto sauce evenly over the lavash bread.

4. Top the sauce with a mixture of your favorite vegetables, such as sliced bell peppers, cherry tomatoes, sliced mushrooms, and sliced red onions.

5. Sprinkle shredded mozzarella cheese or feta cheese over the vegetables.

6. Season with dried oregano, dried basil, salt, and pepper.

7. Bake the lavash pizza in the preheated oven for about 10-12 minutes, or until the cheese is melted and bubbly and the edges of the lavash bread are crispy.

8. Remove it from the oven and let it cool for a minute.

Nutritional information per serving:

Kcal	Carbs	Protein	Fat	Sugar	Fiber
206	21g	11g	8g	7g	4g

DAY 18

Breakfast: Apple-Tahini Toast

 10' 2

Ingredients:

2 slices whole grain bread
2 tablespoons tahini
1 apple, thinly sliced
1 tablespoon honey
1 tablespoon chopped walnuts

1. Toast slices of whole-grain bread until golden and crispy.

2. Spread a generous layer of tahini paste on each slice of toast.

3. Thinly slice a fresh apple and arrange the slices on top of the tahini.

4. Drizzle honey or maple syrup over the apple slices for added sweetness.

5. Sprinkle with a pinch of cinnamon or nutmeg for extra flavor.

6. Serve the apple-tahini toast as a delicious and nutritious breakfast option.

Nutritional information per serving:

Kcal	Carbs	Protein	Fat	Sugar	Fiber
123	17g	4g	6g	10g	3g

Lunch: Cumin Quinoa Pilaf

 25' 2

Ingredients:

1 cup quinoa
2 cups vegetable broth
1 tablespoon olive oil
1 onion, diced
2 cloves garlic, minced
1 teaspoon ground cumin
Salt and pepper to taste
Fresh parsley for garnish

1. Rinse quinoa under cold water to remove any bitterness.

2. In a saucepan, heat olive oil over medium heat.

3. Add diced onions and minced garlic to the saucepan and sauté until fragrant and translucent.

4. Add the rinsed quinoa to the saucepan and toast it for a few minutes, stirring constantly.

5. Pour vegetable broth or water into the saucepan and bring it to a boil.

6. Reduce the heat to low, cover the saucepan, and let the quinoa simmer for about 15-20 minutes, or until the liquid is absorbed and the quinoa is fluffy.

7. In a separate pan, toast cumin seeds until fragrant and lightly browned.

8. Add the toasted cumin seeds to the cooked quinoa and mix well. Season with salt and pepper to taste.

Nutritional information per serving:

Kcal	Carbs	Protein	Fat	Sugar	Fiber
208	32g	7g	7g	2g	4g

Dinner: Lamb Tagine with Couscous and Almonds

 30' 2

Ingredients:

12 ounces lamb, cubed	1 teaspoon ground cinnamon
1 tablespoon olive oil	1 can (10 ounces) diced tomatoes
1 onion, diced	1 cup vegetable broth
2 cloves garlic, minced	1/2 cup dried apricots, chopped
1 teaspoon ground cumin	1/4 cup sliced almonds, toasted
1 teaspoon ground coriander	Cooked couscous for serving

1. In a large pot or tagine, heat olive oil over medium heat.

2. Add diced lamb and cook until browned on all sides.

3. Add chopped onions, minced garlic, and Moroccan spice blend to the pot and sauté for a few minutes until fragrant.

4. Pour vegetable broth or water into the pot until the lamb is covered.

5. Cover the pot and let the lamb simmer over low heat for about 1-2 hours, or until tender.

6. In a separate pot, cook the couscous according to the package instructions.

7. Fluff the cooked couscous with a fork and set aside.

8. In a small pan, toast slivered almonds until golden and fragrant.

9. Once the lamb is tender, stir in cooked couscous and toasted almonds.

10. Taste and adjust the seasoning if needed.

11. Serve the lamb tagine with couscous and almonds hot, garnished with fresh herbs if desired.

Nutritional information per serving:

Kcal	Carbs	Protein	Fat	Sugar	Fiber
244	20g	14g	15g	11g	4g

DAY 19

Breakfast: Tomato and Egg Breakfast Pizza	**Lunch:** Grana Padano Risotto

 25' 2

Ingredients:

1 whole wheat pizza crust	4 eggs
1 cup tomato sauce	¼ cup shredded mozzarella cheese
2 cups baby spinach	Salt and pepper to taste

1. Set the oven temperature according to the instructions on the pizza crust packaging.

2. On a floured surface, roll out the pizza dough to the appropriate thickness.

3. Place the rolled-out dough on a pizza stone or baking sheet.

4. Spread a layer of tomato sauce evenly over the dough.

5. Crack eggs onto the pizza, spacing them evenly apart.

6. Sprinkle grated cheese, such as mozzarella or cheddar, over the eggs.

7. Add your choice of toppings, such as sliced tomatoes, bell peppers, onions, or spinach.

8. Season with salt, pepper, and any desired herbs or spices, such as oregano or basil.

9. Bake in the preheated oven for the time indicated on the pizza crust package.

10. Remove from the oven and let it cool

Nutritional information per serving:

Kcal	Carbs	Protein	Fat	Sugar	Fiber
317	39g	15g	12g	5g	5g

Lunch: Grana Padano Risotto

30' 2

Ingredients:

1 tablespoon olive oil	4 cups vegetable broth
1 onion, diced	1/2 cup grated Grana Padano cheese
2 cloves garlic, minced	Salt and pepper to taste
1 cup Arborio rice	

1. In a large saucepan, heat olive oil over medium heat.

2. Add diced onions and minced garlic to the saucepan and sauté until fragrant and translucent.

3. Add Arborio rice to the saucepan and toast it for a few minutes, stirring constantly.

4. Pour a ladleful of vegetable broth or chicken broth into the saucepan and stir until the liquid is absorbed.

5. Continue adding the broth gradually, stirring frequently, until the rice is cooked al dente (tender but still slightly firm to the bite).

6. Grate Grana Padano cheese and add it to the risotto, stirring until the cheese is melted and the risotto becomes creamy.

8. Serve the Grana Padano risotto hot, garnished with freshly grated cheese and chopped parsley if desired.

Nutritional information per serving:

Kcal	Carbs	Protein	Fat	Sugar	Fiber
276	46g	7g	7g	3g	1g

Dinner: Cheesy Sweet Potato Burgers

 30' 2

Ingredients:

2 medium sweet potatoes, cooked and mashed	1 teaspoon smoked paprika
1 cup cooked quinoa	Salt and pepper to taste
1/2 cup breadcrumbs	Whole wheat burger buns
1/4 cup grated Parmesan cheese	Toppings: lettuce, tomato, onion, pickles, etc.
1/4 cup chopped fresh parsley	

1. Preheat the oven to 400°F (200°C).

2. Peel and grate sweet potatoes using a box grater.

3. In a large mixing bowl, combine the grated sweet potatoes, cooked quinoa, breadcrumbs, grated cheese (such as cheddar or Gouda), minced garlic, chopped parsley, and beaten eggs.

4. Season with salt, pepper, and any desired spices or herbs, such as paprika or cumin.

5. Mix well until all the ingredients are evenly combined.

6. Form the mixture into burger patties of your desired size and thickness.

7. Place the patties on a baking sheet lined with parchment paper.

8. Bake in the preheated oven for about 20-25 minutes, or until the patties are cooked through and golden brown on the outside.

9. While the burgers are baking, prepare any desired burger toppings, such as lettuce, tomato slices, and condiments.

10. Once the burgers are cooked, assemble them with the toppings on your choice of burger buns.

Nutritional information per serving:

Kcal	Carbs	Protein	Fat	Sugar	Fiber
265	50g	10g	4g	9g	7g

DAY 20

Breakfast: Avocado and Egg Toast	**Lunch:** Mint Brown Rice

 15' 2

 30' 2

Ingredients:

2 slices whole wheat bread
1 ripe avocado, mashed

2 eggs, cooked to your preference (fried, poached, or scrambled)
Salt and pepper to taste

1. Toast your choice of bread slices until they are golden and crispy.

2. Cut one avocado in half and remove the pit while the bread is browning. Put the avocado flesh in a small dish by scooping it out.

3. Use a fork to mash the avocado to the desired smoothness.

4. Season the mashed avocado with salt, pepper, and any desired additional spices or herbs, such as chili flakes or cilantro.

5. In a separate pan, fry or poach an egg to your preferred doneness.

6. After the bread has been lightly toasted, generously cover each piece with mashed avocado.

7. Place the cooked egg on top of the avocado spread. Season the egg with salt, pepper, and any desired spices or herbs.

8. Garnish with additional toppings such as sliced tomatoes, microgreens, or crumbled feta

Nutritional information per serving:

Kcal	Carbs	Protein	Fat	Sugar	Fiber
111	9g	5g	7g	1g	3g

Ingredients:

1 cup brown rice
2 cups water
¼ cup chopped fresh mint leaves

2 tablespoons lemon juice
Salt to taste

1. Rinse 1 cup of brown rice under cold water to remove any excess starch.

2. In a saucepan, combine the rinsed rice and 2 cups of water or vegetable broth.

3. Over high heat, bring the mixture to a boil.

4. Lower the heat to a low setting, put a lid on the pan, and let the rice simmer for 45 to 50 minutes, or until it is soft and the liquid has been absorbed.

5. Chop some fresh mint leaves into fine pieces while the rice is cooking. Use a fork to fluff the rice when it has finished cooking.

6. Add the chopped mint leaves to the cooked rice and mix well to distribute the mint flavor.

7. Season the rice with salt and pepper to taste.

8. Optional: Drizzle with a little bit of olive oil and sprinkle with lemon zest for extra freshness.

Nutritional information per serving:

Kcal	Carbs	Protein	Fat	Sugar	Fiber
172	36g	4g	2g	1g	2g

Dinner: Cauliflower Rice Risotto with Mushrooms

 25' 2

Ingredients:

1 medium cauliflower, grated into rice-like pieces	2 cloves garlic, minced
1 tablespoon olive oil	1/4 cup vegetable broth
1 onion, finely chopped	1/4 cup grated Parmesan cheese
8 ounces mushrooms, sliced	Salt and pepper to taste

1. Separate florets from a medium-sized cauliflower.

2. Put the cauliflower florets in a food processor, and pulse them until they resemble grains of rice.

3. Bring olive oil to a simmer in a big saucepan.

4. Add the mushrooms in slices and cook them in the skillet until they release moisture and soften.

5. Stir in the garlic powder and simmer for one more minute, or until aromatic.

6. Stir the mushrooms, garlic, and cauliflower rice together in the skillet.

7. Pour in vegetable broth or chicken broth, enough to cover the cauliflower rice.

8. Bring the mixture to a simmer and cook for about 5-7 minutes, stirring occasionally, until the cauliflower rice is tender.

9. Stir in grated Parmesan cheese, chopped fresh parsley, and season with salt and pepper to taste.

10. Optional: Add a squeeze of lemon juice or a splash of white wine for extra flavor.

11. Serve the cauliflower rice risotto with mushrooms hot, garnished with additional grated Parmesan cheese and a sprinkle of parsley.

Nutritional information per serving:

Kcal	Carbs	Protein	Fat	Sugar	Fiber
94	9g	5g	5g	4g	3g

DAY 21

Breakfast: Tropical Paradise Smoothie Bowl

 10' 2

Ingredients:

2 ripe mangoes, peeled and diced
1 cup pineapple chunks
1 cup coconut milk

1 ripe banana
¼ cup granola
Sliced bananas and shredded coconut for topping

1. In a blender, combine the mangoes, pineapple chunks, coconut milk, and banana. Blend until smooth and creamy.

2. Pour the smoothie into bowls and top with granola, sliced bananas, and shredded coconut.

Nutritional Information (per serving):

Kcal	Carbs	Protein	Fat	Sugar	Fiber
280	39g	3g	16g	30g	5g

Lunch: Mediterranean Lemon Garlic Pasta

 15' 2

Ingredients:

6 ounces whole wheat spaghetti
2 tablespoons extra virgin olive oil
4 garlic cloves, minced
1 cup cherry tomatoes, halved
1/2 cup Kalamata olives, pitted and halved

1/4 cup chopped fresh parsley
2 tablespoons lemon juice
Salt and pepper to taste
Grated Parmesan cheese (optional)

1. Turn on the fire under the pot and wait for the water to boil. Add the salt and the spaghetti, and cook according to the package instructions until al dente.

2. While the pasta is cooking. Olive oil should be heated in a large pan over medium heat. Add the minced garlic and cook until fragrant, about 1 minute.

3. Include the Kalamata olives and cherry tomatoes in the skillet. Cook the tomatoes for 3 to 4 minutes, or until they start to soften.

4. Add the cooked spaghetti, lemon juice, and fresh parsley. To thoroughly incorporate all the ingredients, stir well. To taste, add salt and pepper to the food.

5. For an additional taste boost, serve with grated Parmesan cheese on top.

Nutritional Information (per serving):

Kcal	Carbs	Protein	Fat	Sugar	Fiber
327	46g	8g	13g	2g	7g

Dinner: Baked Salmon with Basil and Tomato

 25' 2

Ingredients:

4 salmon fillets
2 tablespoons olive oil
2 cloves garlic, minced

1 cup cherry tomatoes, halved
1/4 cup fresh basil leaves, chopped
Salt and pepper

1. Preheat the oven to 400°F (200°C).

2. Place salmon fillets on a baking sheet lined with parchment paper.

3. Drizzle the salmon fillets with olive oil and season with salt and pepper.

4. In a small bowl, mix together minced garlic, chopped fresh basil, and diced tomatoes.

5. Spoon the tomato-basil mixture over the salmon fillets, evenly distributing it.

6. Optional: Drizzle the salmon with a squeeze of lemon juice for extra brightness.

7. Bake the salmon for 12 to 15 minutes in a preheated oven, or until it is cooked through and flakes readily with a fork.

8. Remove the salmon from the oven and let it rest for a few minutes. Serve with basil and tomato sauce, garnished with additional fresh basil leaves.

Nutritional information per serving:

Kcal	Carbs	Protein	Fat	Sugar	Fiber
300	2g	25g	21g	1g	1g

DAY 22

Breakfast: Creamy Vanilla Oatmeal

 15'   *2*

Ingredients:

1 cup rolled oats
2 cups almond milk
(or any preferred
milk)
1 tablespoon honey

1 teaspoon vanilla
extract
Fresh berries for
topping

1. Bring water to a boil in a saucepan.

2. Include rolled oats and lower the heat.

3. Prepare the oats as directed on the package, stirring periodically.

4. Once the oats are cooked, remove the saucepan from the heat.

5. Stir in vanilla extract, a pinch of salt, and a drizzle of honey or maple syrup for sweetness.

6. Optional: Add a splash of milk or cream for a creamier texture.

7. Serve the creamy vanilla oatmeal in bowls and top with your choice of sliced fruits, nuts, or a sprinkle of cinnamon.

Nutritional information per serving:

Kcal	Carbs	Protein	Fat	Sugar	Fiber
166	30g	4g	3g	14g	4g

Lunch: Farro Salad with Roasted Vegetables

 30'   *2*

Ingredients:

1 cup farro
2 cups vegetable
broth
1 medium zucchini,
diced
1 red bell pepper,
diced
1 yellow bell pepper,
diced
1 cup cherry tomatoes

¼ cup chopped fresh
basil
2 tablespoons extra-
virgin olive oil
2 tablespoons
balsamic vinegar
Salt and pepper to
taste

1. Rinse the farro under cold water and drain.

2. In a saucepan, bring the vegetable broth to a boil.

3. Add the farro to the boiling broth, reduce the heat to low, cover the pan, and let it simmer for 20-25 minutes, or until the farro is tender but still chewy.

4. Meanwhile, preheat the oven to 400°F (200°C).

5. In a baking dish, combine the diced zucchini, diced red and yellow bell peppers, and cherry tomatoes.

6. Drizzle the vegetables with olive oil, balsamic vinegar, salt, and pepper. Toss to coat.

7. Roast the vegetables in the preheated oven for 15-20 minutes, or until they are tender and slightly caramelized.

8. Once the farro is cooked, drain any excess liquid and transfer it to a large mixing bowl.

Nutritional Information (per serving):

Kcal	Carbs	Protein	Fat	Sugar	Fiber
251	39g	6g	8g	6g	5g

Dinner: Spiced Roast Chicken

 35'   2

Ingredients:

4 chicken drumsticks	1/2 teaspoon cumin
1 tablespoon olive oil	1/2 teaspoon garlic
1 teaspoon paprika	powder
	Salt and pepper to
	taste

1. Preheat the oven to 425°F (220°C).

2. In a small bowl, mix together ground cumin, paprika, garlic powder, salt, and pepper to create a spice rub.

3. Place chicken pieces (such as drumsticks or bone-in chicken breasts) on a baking sheet lined with parchment paper.

4. Rub the spice mixture all over the chicken, ensuring it is evenly coated.

5. Drizzle olive oil over the chicken pieces.

6. Optional: Squeeze fresh lemon juice over the chicken for added tanginess.

7. Roast the chicken in the preheated oven for about 30-40 minutes, or until the internal temperature reaches 165°F (74°C) and the skin is golden and crispy.

8. Remove the chicken from the oven and let it rest for a few minutes before serving.

9. Serve the spiced roast chicken hot, accompanied by your choice of roasted vegetables, steamed rice, or a fresh salad.

Nutritional information per serving:

Kcal	Carbs	Protein	Fat	Sugar	Fiber
170	1g	15g	12g	0g	1g

DAY 23

Breakfast: Mediterranean Citrus Smoothie

 10' 2

Ingredients:

2 oranges, peeled and segmented	1 tablespoon fresh mint leaves
1 grapefruit, peeled and segmented	1 cup ice cubes

1. In a blender, combine the oranges, grapefruit, fresh mint leaves, and ice cubes. Blend until smooth and frothy.

Nutritional Information (per serving):

Kcal	Carbs	Protein	Fat	Sugar	Fiber
33	8g	1g	0g	6g	1g

Lunch: Bulgur Salad with Chickpeas and Herbs

 15' 2

Ingredients:

1 cup bulgur	¼ cup diced red onion
2 cups boiling water	¼ cup diced cucumber
1 can (10 ounce) chickpeas, drained and rinsed	2 tablespoons lemon juice
½ cup chopped fresh parsley	2 tablespoons extra-virgin olive oil
¼ cup chopped fresh mint leaves	Salt and pepper to taste

1. Pour the boiling water over the bulgur that has been placed in a heatproof basin.

2. Cover the bowl with a lid or plastic wrap and let the bulgur soak for 15-20 minutes, or until it is tender and has absorbed the water. Fluff the bulgur with a fork and let it cool.

4. In a large mixing bowl, combine the cooked bulgur, chickpeas, chopped parsley, chopped mint leaves, diced red onion, and cucumber.

5. Combine the lemon juice, olive oil, salt, and pepper in a small bowl.

6. Add the dressing and gently mix to combine. Serve at room temperature.

Nutritional Information (per serving):

Kcal	Carbs	Protein	Fat	Sugar	Fiber
286	43g	9g	9g	3g	9g

Dinner: Lemony Shrimp with Orzo Salad

 25' 2

Ingredients:

12 ounces shrimp, peeled and deveined	2 cups cooked orzo pasta
2 cloves garlic, minced	1 cup cherry tomatoes, halved
Zest and juice of 1 lemon	1/2 cup chopped fresh parsley
2 tablespoons olive oil	1/4 cup crumbled feta cheese
Salt and pepper to taste	

1. Prepare orzo pasta as directed on the packet until it is al dente.

2. In a large bowl, combine cooked orzo, cooked shrimp (peeled and deveined), halved cherry tomatoes, diced cucumbers, chopped fresh dill, and crumbled feta cheese.

3. In a separate small bowl, whisk together lemon juice, olive oil, minced garlic, salt, and pepper to create a tangy dressing.

4. After adding the dressing, mix the orzo salad thoroughly to evenly cover all the ingredients.

Nutritional information per serving:

Kcal	Carbs	Protein	Fat	Sugar	Fiber
309	25g	30g	11g	2g	3g

DAY 24

Breakfast: Healthy Chia Pudding

 5' + overnight chilling   2

Ingredients:

¼ cup chia seeds
1 cup unsweetened
almond milk
1 tablespoon honey or
maple syrup

½ teaspoon vanilla
extract
Fresh berries for
topping

1. Combine chia seeds, your preferred milk (like almond or coconut milk), and your preferred sweetener (like honey or maple syrup) in a dish.

2. Make sure the chia seeds are well-coated with the liquid by giving them a good stir.

3. Stir the mixture once more to avoid clumping after letting it settle for about 5 minutes.

4. To let the chia seeds to absorb the liquid and thicken, cover the bowl and place it in the refrigerator for at least 4 hours or overnight.

5. Stir the chia pudding thoroughly to remove any clumps before serving.

6. To enhance flavor and texture, top with fresh fruit, nuts, or a dusting of cinnamon.

Nutritional information per serving:

Kcal	Carbs	Protein	Fat	Sugar	Fiber
90	11g	3g	5g	5g	5g

Lunch: Lentil and Vegetable Curry Stew

 30'   2

Ingredients:

1 cup dry lentils,
rinsed and drained
1 tablespoon olive oil
1 onion, diced
2 cloves garlic,
minced
1 tablespoon curry
powder
1 teaspoon ground
cumin

1 teaspoon ground
turmeric
1 can diced tomatoes
2 cups vegetable
broth
2 cups chopped
vegetables (such as
carrots, bell peppers,
and zucchini)
Salt and pepper to
taste

1. Heat olive oil in a large pot or Dutch oven over medium heat.

2. Add diced onion, minced garlic, and grated ginger to the pot.

3. Sauté until the onions are translucent and fragrant.

4. Add your choice of chopped vegetables to the pot. Stir in curry powder, ground cumin, ground coriander, and chili.

5. Cook for a few minutes to toast the spices and coat the vegetables.

6. Pour vegetable broth and canned diced tomatoes into the pot. Add the cooked lentils and stir well to combine.

7. Bring the mixture to a boil, then reduce the heat and let it simmer for about 20-25 minutes

Nutritional information per serving:

Kcal	Carbs	Protein	Fat	Sugar	Fiber
270	45g	15g	5g	6g	8g

Dinner: Grilled Chicken and Zucchini Kebabs

 20'   *2*

Ingredients:

12 ounces boneless, skinless chicken breasts, cut into chunks	2 tablespoons lemon juice
2 zucchini, cut into chunks	2 cloves garlic, minced
2 tablespoons olive oil	1 teaspoon dried oregano
	Salt and pepper to taste

1. Preheat the grill to medium-high heat.

2. Cut boneless, skinless chicken breasts into chunks and place them in a bowl.

3. Drizzle olive oil over the chicken and add minced garlic, dried oregano, lemon zest, salt, and pepper.

4. Toss the chicken to coat it evenly with the marinade.

5. Cut zucchini into thick slices and toss them in olive oil, salt, and pepper.

6. Thread the marinated chicken and zucchini slices onto skewers, alternating between them.

7. Place the kebabs on the preheated grill and cook for about 8-10 minutes, turning occasionally, until the chicken is cooked through and the zucchini is tender and slightly charred.

8. Remove the kebabs from the grill and let them rest for a few minutes.

9. Serve the grilled chicken and zucchini kebabs with a side of couscous or a fresh salad.

Nutritional information per serving:

Kcal	Carbs	Protein	Fat	Sugar	Fiber
220	5g	27g	11g	3g	2g

DAY 25

Breakfast: Feta and Spinach Frittata

 25' 2

Ingredients:

6 large eggs	¼ cup diced red bell
½ cup crumbled feta	pepper
cheese	¼ cup diced red
1 cup fresh spinach,	onion
chopped	Salt and pepper to
	taste

1. Preheat the oven to 350°F (175°C).

2. In a mixing bowl, whisk together eggs, crumbled feta cheese, chopped spinach, diced tomatoes, minced garlic, and dried oregano.

3. Season with salt and pepper to taste.

4. Heat a non-stick ovenproof skillet over medium heat and add olive oil.

5. Pour the egg mixture into the skillet and cook for a few minutes until the edges start to set.

6. Transfer the skillet to the preheated oven and bake for about 12-15 minutes, or until the frittata is set and slightly golden on top.

7. Remove it from the oven and let it cool slightly before slicing.

8. Serve the feta and spinach frittata warm or at room temperature.

Nutritional information per serving:

Kcal	Carbs	Protein	Fat	Sugar	Fiber
165	3g	12g	12g	1g	1g

Lunch: Wild Rice, Celery, and Cauliflower Pilaf

 20' 2

Ingredients:

1 cup cooked wild rice	2 tablespoons lemon
1 cup cauliflower	juice
florets, finely chopped	1 tablespoon chopped
1/2 cup diced celery	fresh parsley
2 tablespoons olive oil	Salt and pepper to
	taste

1. Cook wild rice according to package instructions until tender.

2. Heat olive oil in a large skillet over medium heat.

3. Add diced onion and sliced celery to the skillet.

4. Sauté until the vegetables are softened.

5. Add minced garlic, cauliflower florets, and a pinch of dried thyme.

6. Stir and cook for a few minutes until the cauliflower starts to soften.

7. Stir in the cooked wild rice and season with salt and pepper. Add vegetable broth and bring the mixture to a simmer.

8. Cover the skillet and let it cook for about 10-15 minutes until the cauliflower is tender and the flavors are well combined.

Nutritional information per serving:

Kcal	Carbs	Protein	Fat	Sugar	Fiber
116	11g	3g	7g	2g	2g

Dinner: Roasted Chicken Thighs With Basmati

 30'   2

Ingredients:

4 bone-in, skin-on
chicken thighs
1 cup basmati rice
2 cups chicken broth
2 tablespoons olive oil

1 teaspoon paprika
1 teaspoon dried
thyme
Salt and pepper to
taste

1. Set the oven temperature to 425°F (220°C).

2. In a baking dish, arrange the chicken thighs and sprinkle them with salt, pepper, dried rosemary, and garlic powder.

3. Sprinkle olive oil over the chicken and season the flesh by rubbing it in.

4. To enhance flavor, place lemon slices on top of the chicken thighs.

5. In a separate pot, cook basmati rice according to package instructions.

6. Once the rice is cooked, fluff it with a fork and season it with salt and a squeeze of lemon juice.

7. Place the baking dish with the chicken thighs in the preheated oven and roast for about 25-30 minutes until the chicken is cooked through and the skin is crispy.

8. Remove the chicken from the oven and let it rest for a few minutes.

9. Serve the roasted chicken thighs with a side of fluffy basmati rice and steamed vegetables.

Nutritional information per serving:

Kcal	Carbs	Protein	Fat	Sugar	Fiber
501	33g	25g	30g	1g	1g

DAY 26

Breakfast: Protein-Packed Almond Butter Smoothie

 10'   2

Ingredients:

2 tablespoons almond butter
1 cup Greek yogurt
1 ripe banana

1 cup almond milk
½ teaspoon cinnamon
Ice cubes (optional)

1. In a blender, combine the almond butter, Greek yogurt, banana, almond milk, and cinnamon.

2. Blend until creamy and smooth. For a cold smoothie, if preferred, add ice cubes and combine one more.

Nutritional Information (per serving):

Kcal	Carbs	Protein	Fat	Sugar	Fiber
150	14g	6g	7g	10g	2g

Lunch: Seashell Pasta with Shrimp and Cherry Tomatoes

 25'   2

Ingredients

1 tablespoon extra-virgin olive oil
12 ounces shrimp, deveined shells removed
2 cloves garlic, chopped, or to taste

1/2 cup white cooking wine
15/20 cherry tomatoes
6 ounces - small seashell pasta

1. First, wash the inside and outside of the shrimp in warm water and remove the heads, legs, and carapace (the shell).

2. Cut into the back of the shrimp with a small knife or toothpick and remove the intestines by pulling gently. Rinse and set aside

3. Heat the oil in a skillet over low heat and brown the garlic for about 2 minutes. Add the cherry tomatoes, cut into 4 pieces, and cook for another 2 minutes.

4. Add the wine and raise the heat to let the alcohol evaporate

5. In another pot, boil water. As soon as the water boils, add the salt and toss in the pasta

6. Taste the pasta; it must be al dente. Drain it and pour it into the shrimp. Stir and cook for 5 minutes more, or until the desired consistency is reached. Serve and enjoy!

Nutritional Information (per serving):

Kcal	Carbs	Protein	Fat	Sugar	Fiber
324	45g	20g	6g	2g	2g

Dinner: Zucchini Fritters

 25' 2

Ingredients:

2 medium zucchini, grated
1/2 cup breadcrumbs
1/4 cup grated Parmesan cheese
1/4 cup chopped fresh parsley
2 cloves garlic, minced

1/4 teaspoon salt
1/4 teaspoon black pepper
1 large egg, beaten
2 tablespoons olive oil

1. Grate zucchini using a box grater or a food processor.

2. Place the grated zucchini in a colander and sprinkle with salt.Let the zucchini sit for about 10 minutes to draw out the excess moisture.

3. Squeeze out the excess liquid from the zucchini using your hands or a clean kitchen towel.

4. Transfer the grated and drained zucchini to a mixing bowl.

5. Add breadcrumbs, grated Parmesan cheese, minced garlic, chopped fresh parsley, beaten eggs, and a pinch of black pepper.

6. Mix well until all the ingredients are evenly combined.

7. Heat olive oil in a large skillet over medium heat.

8. Scoop about 1/4 cup of the zucchini mixture and form it into a patty shape.

9. Place the zucchini fritters in the hot skillet and cook for about 2-3 minutes per side until golden brown and crispy.

10. Repeat the process with the remaining zucchini mixture, adding more oil to the skillet as needed.

11. Once cooked, transfer the zucchini fritters to a paper towel-lined plate to absorb any excess oil.

Nutritional information per serving:

Kcal	Carbs	Protein	Fat	Sugar	Fiber
173	14g	7g	12g	4g	2g

DAY 27

Breakfast: Mediterranean Shakshuka

 15' 2

Ingredients:

2 tablespoons olive oil	1 teaspoon cumin
½ onion, thinly sliced	1 teaspoon paprika
2 cloves garlic, minced	½ teaspoon chili flakes (optional)
1 red bell pepper, thinly sliced	Salt and pepper to taste
1 can (400g) diced tomatoes	4-6 large eggs
	Fresh parsley for garnish

1. Heat olive oil in a skillet over medium heat.

2. Add the sliced onions and minced garlic to the skillet. Sauté until the onions are translucent.

3. Add the red bell pepper slices to the skillet and cook for a few minutes until they start to soften.

4. Pour in the diced tomatoes, cumin, paprika, and chili flakes (if using). Season with salt and pepper.

5. Simmer the tomato mixture for about 10 minutes until the flavors meld together.

6. Create small wells in the sauce and crack the eggs into the wells.

7. Cover the skillet and cook for about 5-7 minutes

Nutritional Information (per serving):

Kcal	Carbs	Protein	Fat	Sugar	Fiber
165	6g	7g	12g	1g	1g

Lunch: Greek Salad with Lemon-Herb Dressing

 15' 2

Ingredients:

2 cups mixed salad greens	1/4 cup Kalamata olives, pitted
1/2 cucumber, diced	1/4 cup crumbled feta cheese
1/2 red bell pepper, diced	2 tablespoons fresh dill, chopped
1/2 yellow bell pepper, diced	2 tablespoons fresh parsley, chopped
1/4 red onion, thinly sliced	Juice of 1 lemon
1 cup cherry tomatoes, halved	2 tablespoons extra-virgin olive oil
	Salt and pepper to taste

1. In a large salad bowl, combine the mixed salad greens, cucumber, bell peppers, red onion, cherry tomatoes, Kalamata olives, feta cheese, dill, and parsley.

2. In a small bowl, whisk together the lemon juice, olive oil, salt, and pepper to make the dressing.

3. Drizzle the dressing over the salad and toss gently to coat all the ingredients.

Nutritional Information per Serving:

Kcal	Carbs	Protein	Fat	Sugar	Fiber
103	6g	3g	11g	2g	1g

Dinner: Pan-Seared Pompano Fish and Black Olive

 30'   2

Ingredients:

4 pompano fish fillet   1/8 teaspoon sea salt
2 tablespoons extra   1/8 teaspoon ground
virgin olive oil   black pepper Garnish
2 tablespoons capers   4 slices lemon
2 tablespoons black
olives

1. On a skillet, heat the oil over medium for 3 minutes.

2. Coat the fish with oil. Place on the skillet and cook on high for 3 minutes.

3. Sprinkle with capers, olives salt, and pepper.

4. Turn the fish over and cook for 5 more min. or until golden brown and no longer translucent.

5. Transfer to the plates and decorate with the garnishing ingredients.

Nutritional Information (per serving):

Kcal	Carbs	Protein	Fat	Sugar	Fiber
315	2g	27g	23g	0g	0g

DAY 28

Breakfast: Egg Bake

 35' 2

Ingredients:

6 large eggs
1 cup milk
1 cup diced bell peppers
1 cup diced onions

1 cup diced mushrooms
1 cup shredded cheddar cheese
Salt and pepper to taste

1. Preheat your oven to the specified temperature according to the recipe.

2. In a mixing bowl, whisk together eggs, milk, salt, pepper, and any additional seasonings or ingredients specified in the recipe.

3. Grease a baking dish or line it with parchment paper. Pour the egg mixture into the baking dish, spreading it evenly. Add any vegetables, cheese, or other toppings as directed in the recipe.

4. Place the baking dish in the preheated oven and bake for the specified time, or until the eggs are set and the top is lightly golden.

5. Once cooked, remove the egg bake from the oven and let it cool for a few minutes before slicing and serving.

Nutritional information per serving:

Kcal	Carbs	Protein	Fat	Sugar	Fiber
323	12g	22g	21g	7g	1g

Lunch: Roasted Ratatouille Pasta

 35' 2

Ingredients:

6 ounces whole wheat penne pasta
1 small eggplant, diced
1 zucchini, diced
1 yellow squash, diced
1 red bell pepper, diced
1 small onion, diced

2 cloves garlic, minced
2 tablespoons olive oil
1 teaspoon dried Italian seasoning
Salt and pepper to taste
Grated Parmesan cheese for serving

1. Preheat your oven to the specified temperature according to the recipe.

2. Chop vegetables such as eggplant, zucchini, bell peppers, and onions into bite-sized pieces.

3. Place the chopped vegetables in a large baking dish.

4. Drizzle olive oil over the vegetables and sprinkle with salt, pepper, and any desired herbs or seasonings.

5. Toss the vegetables to coat them evenly in the oil and seasonings.

6. Place the baking dish in the preheated oven, and roast the vegetables until they are tender and slightly caramelized.

7. While the vegetables are roasting, cook the pasta according to package instructions until al dente.

8. Drain the cooked pasta and transfer it to a large serving bowl with the vegetables.

Nutritional information per serving:

Kcal	Carbs	Protein	Fat	Sugar	Fiber
312	52g	11g	10g	8g	9g

Dinner: Grilled Vegetable Skewers

 30'   2

Ingredients:

1 zucchini, sliced into rounds	2 tablespoons olive oil
1 yellow squash, sliced into rounds	2 tablespoons balsamic vinegar
1 red bell pepper, cut into chunks	2 cloves garlic, minced
1 red onion, cut into chunks	1 teaspoon dried Italian seasoning
8 cherry tomatoes	Salt and pepper to taste

1. Preheat your grill to medium-high heat.

2. Prepare the vegetables by cutting them into chunks or slices, ensuring they are all roughly the same size for even cooking.

3. To avoid scorching, immerse wooden skewers in water for about 30 minutes. Thread the prepared vegetables onto the skewers, alternating between different vegetables for variety.

4. Brush the vegetable skewers with olive oil and season with salt, pepper, and any desired herbs or spices.

5. Place the skewers on the preheated grill and cook for a few minutes on each side until the vegetables are tender and lightly charred.

6. Keep an eye on the skewers and rotate them as needed to ensure even cooking.

7. Once the vegetables are grilled to your desired doneness, remove them from the grill and transfer them to a serving platter.

8. Serve the grilled vegetable skewers as a delicious and colorful dinner option.

Nutritional information per serving:

Kcal	Carbs	Protein	Fat	Sugar	Fiber
108	8g	2g	7g	6g	2g

DAY 29

Breakfast: Pumpkin Pie Parfait

 10' 2

Ingredients:

1 cup canned pumpkin puree	1 teaspoon pumpkin pie spice
1 cup Greek yogurt	1/2 cup granola
2 tablespoons honey	1/4 cup chopped pecans

1. In a bowl or glass, layer pumpkin puree, Greek yogurt, and granola.

2. Sprinkle cinnamon and nutmeg on top for added flavor.

3. Repeat the layers until the bowl or glass is filled, ending with a dollop of Greek yogurt on top.

4. Optionally, garnish with a sprinkle of granola or a drizzle of honey.

5. Serve the pumpkin pie parfait chilled.

Nutritional information per serving:

Kcal	Carbs	Protein	Fat	Sugar	Fiber
212	28g	7g	9g	16g	4g

Lunch: Bean and Veggie Pasta

 20' 2

Ingredients

6 ounces whole wheat penne pasta	1/4 cup chopped fresh basil
1 can (7 ounces) cannellini beans, rinsed and drained	2 tablespoons extra virgin olive oil
1 cup cherry tomatoes, halved	2 tablespoons lemon juice
1 cup baby spinach	2 cloves garlic, minced
	Salt and pepper

1. Turn on the fire under the pot and wait for the water to boil. Add the salt and the penne, and cook according to the package instructions until al dente.

2. While the pasta is cooking. In a large skillet, heat olive oil over medium heat.

3. Add minced garlic and diced onion to the skillet, sautéing until fragrant and the onion is translucent.

4. Add chopped vegetables such as bell peppers, zucchini, and cherry tomatoes to the skillet.

5. Sauté the vegetables until they are tender-crisp. Drain and rinse a can of beans (such as cannellini or kidney beans) and add them to the skillet.

6. Season the mixture with salt, pepper, and any desired herbs or spices. Add the cooked pasta to the skillet and toss everything together until well combined.

7. Cook for an additional minute or two to heat the pasta through. Serve with Parmesan cheese

Nutritional information per serving:

Kcal	Carbs	Protein	Fat	Sugar	Fiber
344	54g	13g	9g	3g	11g

Dinner: Sautéed Green Beans with Tomatoes

 15'   ⊗ 2

Ingredients:

12 ounces green beans, trimmed	2 cloves garlic, minced
1 pint cherry tomatoes, halved	1 teaspoon dried Italian seasoning
2 tablespoons olive oil	Salt and pepper to taste

1. Trim the ends off the green beans and wash them thoroughly.

2. Heat olive oil in a large skillet over medium heat.

3. Add minced garlic to the skillet and sauté until fragrant.

4. Add the green beans to the skillet and sauté for a few minutes until they start to soften.

5. Add diced tomatoes to the skillet and continue sautéing until the green beans are tender and the tomatoes are heated through.

6. Season with salt, pepper, and any desired herbs or spices.

7. Cook for an additional minute or two to combine the flavors.

8. Serve the sautéed green beans with tomatoes as a tasty and nutritious side dish.

Nutritional information per serving:

Kcal	Carbs	Protein	Fat	Sugar	Fiber
116	12g	3g	7g	6g	4g

DAY 30

Breakfast: Berry Blast Smoothie

 10' 2

Ingredients:

2 cups mixed berries (strawberries, blueberries, raspberries)
1 cup Greek yogurt

1 cup spinach
1 tablespoon honey
1 cup almond milk

1. In a blender, combine the mixed berries, Greek yogurt, spinach, honey, and almond milk.

2. Blend on high speed until smooth and creamy. Pour into glasses and serve immediately.

Nutritional Information (per serving):

Kcal	Carbs	Protein	Fat	Sugar	Fiber
124	15g	5g	3g	15g	3g

Lunch: Brussels Sprouts Linguine

 25' 2

Ingredients:

6 ounces whole wheat linguine
2 cups Brussels sprouts, trimmed and halved
2 tablespoons olive oil

¼ cup grated Parmesan cheese
¼ cup chopped toasted walnuts
Salt and pepper
2 cloves garlic, minced

1. Turn on the fire under the pot and wait for the water to boil. Add the salt and the linguine, and cook according to the package instructions until al dente.

2. While the pasta is cooking, prepare the Brussels sprouts.

3. Trim the ends of the Brussels sprouts and remove any yellow or damaged outer leaves. Cut the Brussels sprouts into halves or quarters. In a large skillet, heat olive oil over medium heat.

4. Add minced garlic and red pepper flakes, and sauté for a minute until fragrant.

5. Add the Brussels sprouts to the skillet and cook, stirring occasionally, until they are tender and slightly caramelized. Season with salt and pepper to taste.

6. Drain the cooked linguine and add it to the skillet with the Brussels sprouts.

7. Sprinkle some grated Parmesan cheese

Nutritional information per serving:

Kcal	Carbs	Protein	Fat	Sugar	Fiber
354	47g	12g	15g	2g	7g

Dinner: Chicken Breast Hummus and Feta Cheese

 20' 2

Ingredients:

Tacos: 2 chicken breasts (brined in 2 tbsp. of salt and 2 cups of water)
4 tortilla wraps bread
2 tomatoes, diced
1 large cucumber, peeled and diced
1 small yellow onion, diced
2 tablespoons white wine vinegar

1/4 cup extra virgin olive oil
1/2 teaspoon sea salt
1/2 teaspoon minced sweet Italian pepper
1 container hummus
1 1/2 cups shredded lettuce
1 can artichoke hearts, drained
sliced green olives
1/2 cup feta cheese, crumbled

1. Soak the meat in 2 cups of water and 2 tbsp. of saltwater. Pan-fry or grill until the juices run clear and the meat registers an internal temperature. of 155 degrees F.

2. Mix all of the vegetable ingredients. Layer the pita wrap with the topping ingredients, meat, and vegetable ingredients.

Nutritional information per serving

Kcal	Carbs	Protein	Fat	Sugar	Fiber
600	62g	22g	32g	4g	15g

Notes on recipes in the book: the exact nutritional information may vary depending on the specific brands and quantities of ingredients used. It's always a good idea to refer to the nutritional labels on the products you use for the most accurate information.

CHAPTER 10: *Sustaining the Mediterranean Lifestyle*

Maintaining a Balanced Diet

Maintaining a balanced diet is key to sustaining the Mediterranean lifestyle and reaping its long-term health benefits. Here are some important principles to keep in mind:

1. **Variety is Essential:** Continue to incorporate a wide variety of fruits, vegetables, whole grains, legumes, nuts, seeds, lean proteins, and healthy fats into your meals. Experiment with different ingredients to keep your meals interesting and flavorful.

2. **Portion Control**: While the Mediterranean diet is known for its flexibility, it's important to practice portion control to maintain a healthy weight. Be mindful of your serving sizes and listen to your body's hunger and fullness cues.

3. **Limit Processed Foods**: Minimize your consumption of processed and packaged foods, which are often high in added sugars, unhealthy fats, and sodium. Opt for whole, unprocessed foods as much as possible.

4. **Moderation is Key:** While the Mediterranean diet encourages the consumption of wine and certain indulgences, it's important to enjoy these items in moderation. Balance is the key to maintaining a healthy and sustainable eating pattern.

5. **Stay hydrated.** Don't forget to drink plenty of water throughout the day. Hydration is essential for overall health and wellbeing.

Incorporating Exercise and Physical Activity

Regular exercise and physical activity are crucial components of the Mediterranean lifestyle. Here are some tips to help you incorporate exercise into your daily routine:

1. **Find Activities You Enjoy:** Choose activities that you genuinely enjoy, whether it's brisk walking, cycling, swimming, dancing, or playing a sport. Engaging in activities you love increases the likelihood of sticking with them long-term.

2. **Aim for 150 Minutes per Week**: Strive to accumulate at least 150 minutes of moderate-intensity aerobic activity, such as brisk walking, every week. This can be spread out over several days to fit your schedule.

3. **Strength Training**: Include at least two days a week of strength training activities. This might involve utilizing resistance bands, lifting weights, or performing bodyweight workouts. Muscle mass is essential for maintaining and gaining strength, as well as for a healthy body composition and metabolism.

4. **Stay Active** Throughout the Day: Look for opportunities to stay active throughout the day, such as taking the stairs instead of the elevator, parking farther away from your destination, or going for short walks during breaks.

Mindful Eating and Portion Control

Mindful eating and portion control play a significant role in the Mediterranean lifestyle. Here's how you can incorporate these practices into your daily life:

1. **Slow Down and Savor**: Take the time to enjoy your meals and pay attention to the flavors, textures, and aromas of the food. Eating slowly and mindfully can help you better recognize your body's hunger and fullness cues.

2. **2. Use Smaller Plates and Bowls:** To regulate portion proportions, choose smaller plates and bowls. This might deceive your brain into thinking you need less food to feel full.

3. **Listen to Your Body:** Eat when you're hungry and stop when you're pleasantly full. 3. Listen to Your Body. Never eat while you're bored or feeling upset. Recognize the difference between emotional and bodily hunger.

4. **Practice Mindful Snacking:** If you snack between meals, choose nutritious options such as fruits, vegetables, nuts, or yogurt. Be mindful of portion sizes even when snacking.

Staying Motivated and Overcoming Challenges

Maintaining a Mediterranean lifestyle can sometimes be challenging. Here are some strategies to help you stay motivated and overcome obstacles:

1. **Set practical Goals:** Make sure your goals are both attainable and practical.

2. **Find Support:** Seek support from family, friends, or a community of like-minded individuals who are also following a Mediterranean lifestyle. Share your challenges, successes, and experiences with them.

3. **Keep a Food and Activity Journal:** Maintain a journal to track your meals, exercise, and emotions. This can help you identify patterns, track progress, and stay accountable.

4. **Plan Ahead**: Plan your meals and snacks in advance and make a shopping list to ensure you have the necessary ingredients on hand. This can help you make healthier choices and avoid impulsive food decisions.

5. **Reward Yourself**: Celebrate your milestones and successes along the way. Treat yourself to non-food rewards such as a relaxing massage, a new book, or a day trip to keep yourself motivated.

Celebrating Progress and Long-Term Success

Celebrating your progress and maintaining long-term success is an essential part of the Mediterranean lifestyle. Here are some ways to celebrate your achievements:

1. **Reflect on Your Journey:** Take the time to reflect on how far you've come and the positive changes you've made. Acknowledge your efforts and the impact they've had on your health and wellbeing.

2. **Share Your Success**: Share your Mediterranean lifestyle journey with others. Inspire and motivate those around you to embrace healthier habits and join you on this path to better health.

3. **Try New Recipes and Foods**: Continue to explore new recipes, ingredients, and flavors to keep your meals exciting and diverse. Embrace the culinary traditions of the Mediterranean region and incorporate them into your everyday life.

4. **Stay Informed**: Stay up-to-date with the latest research and information on the Mediterranean lifestyle. This will help you reinforce your knowledge and make informed decisions about your health.

Remember, sustaining the Mediterranean lifestyle is a lifelong commitment to health and wellbeing. Embrace the principles of balance, moderation, and enjoyment and let them become a natural part of your everyday life.

Appendix:

Icons Recipe:

Preparation Time

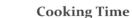
Cooking Time

Marinating Time

Serves

Measurement Conversion Chart

VOLUME EQUIVALENTS(DRY)

US STANDARD	METRIC (APPROXIMATE)
1/8 teaspoon	0.5 mL
1/4 teaspoon	1 mL
1/2 teaspoon	2 mL
3/4 teaspoon	4 mL
1 teaspoon	5 mL
1 tablespoon	15 mL
1/4 cup	59 mL
1/2 cup	118 mL
3/4 cup	177 mL
1 cup	235 mL
2 cups	475 mL
3 cups	700 mL
4 cups	1 L

VOLUME EQUIVALENTS(LIQUID)

US STANDARD	US STANDARD (OUNCES)	METRIC (APPROXIMATE)
2 tablespoons	1 fl.oz.	30 mL
1/4 cup	2 fl.oz.	60 mL
1/2 cup	4 fl.oz.	120 mL
1 cup	8 fl.oz.	240 mL
1 1/2 cup	12 fl.oz.	355 mL
2 cups or 1 pint	16 fl.oz.	475 mL
4 cups or 1 quart	32 fl.oz.	1 L
1 gallon	128 fl.oz.	4 L

TEMPERATURES EQUIVALENTS

FAHRENHEIT(F)	CELSIUS(C) (APPROXIMATE)
225 °F	107 °C
250 °F	120 °C
275 °F	135 °C
300 °F	150 °C
325 °F	160 °C
350 °F	180 °C
375 °F	190 °C
400 °F	205 °C
425 °F	220 °C
450 °F	235 °C
475 °F	245 °C
500 °F	260 °C

WEIGHT EQUIVALENTS

US STANDARD	METRIC (APPROXIMATE)
1 ounce	28 g
2 ounces	57 g
5 ounces	142 g
10 ounces	284 g
15 ounces	425 g
16 ounces (1 pound)	455 g
1.5 pounds	680 g
2 pounds	907 g

Dear Reader,

Congratulations on reaching the end of this journey through the Mediterranean lifestyle! I want to take a moment to express my heartfelt gratitude for choosing this book as your guide. It has been an honor to accompany you on this path toward a healthier, more vibrant life.

Throughout this book, we have explored the richness and beauty of the Mediterranean diet, the importance of physical activity and mindful eating, and the keys to sustaining this lifestyle in the long term. I hope that the knowledge and practical tips shared here have empowered you to make positive changes and embrace a way of living that nurtures both your body and mind.

As you embark on the next chapter of your journey, I encourage you to remember that this is not just a book but a roadmap for life. Embrace the principles of the Mediterranean lifestyle with enthusiasm and adapt them to suit your unique needs and preferences. Remember that it's not about achieving perfection but rather making progress and finding joy in the process.

I want to express my sincere appreciation for your trust and dedication. It is my hope that this book has not only provided valuable information but has also sparked a newfound passion within you. May this knowledge guide you to make choices that enhance your well-being and contribute to a healthier, happier life.

With gratitude and warmest wishes,

Theresa R. Campanella

Leave a Review

As an independent author with a small marketing budget, reviews are my livelihood on this platform. If you enjoyed this book, I'd appreciate it if you could leave your honest feedback.

I read EVERY single review because I love the feedback from MY readers!

Thanks

Made in the USA
Las Vegas, NV
03 September 2023

77033161R00077